FORGET-ME-NOT

G

A Memoir of Anne Bashkiroff's Alzheimer's Crusade

Purdue University Press

West Lafayette, Indiana

Printed in the United States of America.

ISBN-13: 978-1-55753-425-5 (alk. paper)
ISBN-10: 1-55753-425-X

Library of Congress Cataloging-in-Publication Data
Holland, Gail Bernice, 1940-
  [For Sasha, with love]
  Forget-me-not : a memoir of Anne Bashkiroff's Alzheimer's
crusade / Gail Bernice Holland.
      p. cm.
  ISBN-13: 978-1-55753-425-5 (alk. paper) 1. Bashkiroff, Anne.
2. Bashkiroff, Sasha. 3. Alzheimer's disease—Patients—Biography.
4. Brain damage—Patients—Services for—United States. 5. Brain
damage—Patients—Legal status, laws, etc.—United States. I. Title.
  RC523.B3H65 2007
  362.196'8310092–dc22
  [B]
                                                    2006028054

CONTENTS

Acknowledgments

I am grateful to the people who have read and commented on areas of specific expertise: Terence Emmons, professor of history at Stanford University, who was kind enough to review my historical chapters; Dr. William Lynch, who checked the medical information; John Bosshardt, who gave me advice on legal matters concerning brain-damaged victims and their families; and Marian Emr with the National Institute of Aging, who contributed her extensive knowledge about the latest research on Alzheimer's disease. My book praises the work of Family Caregiver Alliance (formerly known as the Family Survival Project), and I would like to thank the staff and board of directors for the help they offered, particularly Karla Griffin, Suzanne Harris, Kathleen Kelly, Gary Lile, Jane Ophuls, and Diana Petty.

I also appreciate the support of Linda Bell, Linda Herbert, and Delores De Vasto, and thank all my friends and family, especially my precious daughter Anya Holland-Barry, for giving me the inspiration to write this book.

Gail Bernice Holland

AUTHOR'S NOTE

I could have written this book in the third person, as the objective journalist reporting this story from my own emotional distance. It took me one day toying with several typewritten pages to know that wouldn't work. By then I knew the only way to tell Anne Bashkiroff's story honestly and with heart was to write this book as if I were Anne Bashkiroff.

To the real Anne Bashkiroff I give my eternal thanks. She allowed me to not just step into her shoes, but into her soul. She showed me more than her tears; she made me understand her story so deeply that my own tears came. She had the courage to admit her anger, her fears, her mistakes, until I knew her faults better than my own. But best of all, she showed me the sunshine—her altruism, love, passion for life, and her determination to achieve justice.

This book was written in the loving memory of a husband, but Anne also wanted to pave the way for the future. She hoped by revealing her mistakes she could warn others not to make the same ones. She hoped her victories would encourage people to risk and reach out for their goals.

During the stretch of time that it took me to complete this book it was an honor to be—if only on paper—Anne Bashkiroff.

Gail Bernice Holland

PROLOGUE

She twists the rubber band around her wrist, and pulls it until it is taut. The band snaps against her skin.

Each time Anne Bashkiroff feels the fear rising she snaps it. Each time she thinks—I can't speak. What am I doing here?—she tugs at the rubber band. She tells herself: If I cause a pain sensation on my wrist, maybe I can forget the nervousness in my head.

Rosalynn Carter sits only twenty feet away from her, at a long polished table set with microphones and glasses of water. A person coughs in the audience, and people shift in their seats, restless from the hours of testimony before the President's Commission on Mental Health.

It is almost noon. Rosalynn Carter announces they have nearly completed the morning agenda, and only have time to recognize a few people from the floor. There are hundreds of people in the audience, and many want to speak.

Earlier Anne was informed she might be one of those chosen to testify. She worries: Supposing my fear of public speaking turns my words into gibberish, and I make a fool of myself in front of the wife of the President of the United States?

Yet Anne's need for public advocacy is even more dominant than her fear of public speaking. It's what pushed her into coming to this San Francisco hotel today, what makes her determined to overcome her nervousness, stand up before strangers, and tell her story.

The first name is called. It's not hers. The second speaker finishes his testimony. To Anne, the room feels as if it's running out of oxygen.

"Anne Bashkiroff."

She hears Rosalynn Carter's soft voice call her name. Anne rises and slowly moves to the microphone.

"Mrs. Carter, members of the commission, friends," she begins. "I am a member of the Family Survival Task Force, working under the auspices of the San Francisco Mental Health Association. I am the wife of a man who has irreversible brain damage caused by presenile dementia, also known as Alzheimer's disease. This means his brain tissues are dying. There is no cure.

"For seven years I was able to take care of my husband at home. I watched over him as his memory deteriorated to where he could no longer tell the time of day, sign his name, or say where he lived. His frustration led to anger and violence. In the end, neither I nor the sitters I hired could cope with him. He had to be placed in a skilled nursing facility for the rest of his life. He will never come home to his young son and me again."

She delivers her prepared lines slowly, allowing time for the words to penetrate. The lights from the TV camera are now on her.

"There are two aspects I wish to address. My first concern is the lack of custodial facilities capable of caring for irreversibly brain-damaged adults.

"My husband was thrown out of eight facilities in three months. Because of this treatment he withdrew into himself and became—as this condition is vulgarly known—a vegetable. He does not deserve this. No one does."

Anne accentuates the phrase "no one does." Her voice, which had been barely audible, all at once becomes strong.

"My second concern is the astronomical cost of long-term custodial care and its effects on the middle-income American. The cost ranges from one thousand dollars per month on up. How many of you here can afford this cost?

"I for one cannot. For the poor there is inadequate care, but there is state and federal monetary support. For the middle-income family there is *nothing*. No private insurance covers custodial care. Neither the state nor the federal government provides monetary support.

"What happens to surviving families? Eventual pauperization, destitution, and destruction. We face an American nightmare. We are neither poor enough to be supported, nor rich enough to survive.

"We do not want to be declared wards of the state. We do not want to become medically indigent in our hour of need. This is not only an indignity, it is not even fiscally sound."

The applause interrupts her.

"We are looking for supplemental assistance from the state and federal governments—and *not* total care with the full cost coming from the tax dollar. As survivors we want to continue working and paying our fair share toward the cost of custodial care for our spouses. We do not want to be punished by the system we uphold, as we have already been punished by fate.

"In closing I ask that just as we recognize veterans of war in our country, we must recognize veterans of life."

The applause is now prolonged.

Anne adds, "I urge that you, Mrs. Carter, together with the members of the commission, give immediate attention to legislating special financial assistance to our families. This is a problem that cannot wait for years. It must be dealt with through special executive action in the best American tradition of helping those who help themselves. Thank you."

PART ONE

Chapter 1

LEST WE FORGET

Strange. Some of my sharpest memories of Sasha go back to a time before I even knew him.

When I married Sasha, I married his past; his past became as vivid to me as the years we had together. Twenty years older than I, Sasha was born in Russia before the Revolution. Throughout our marriage he would tell me stories of his childhood in Samara, Russia, and of the vast upheaval his family suffered during the Revolution, repeating these stories regularly until I could correct him if he deviated to the slightest degree.

Then came Alzheimer's disease, a disease that destroys one's ability to think and remember. As the disease progressed and Sasha forgot recent events, his memory of his boyhood years remained intact. His past, his beloved Samara, was almost the last thing the disease destroyed.

I understood why Sasha's family history was so important to him. I, too, had my own stories to tell of my Russian heritage. We were two people who built a future by honoring the lives we lived before we met.

* * *

3

His full name was Alexander Feodrovich Bashkiroff, but his family called him by his diminutive name—Sasha. Born on the estate of his maternal grandfather, Pavel Juraleff, in the countryside of Samara, Sasha's boyhood was marked by prodigious wealth.

Pavel had made his fortune as a landowner, and Nicholas Bashkiroff, Sasha's paternal grandfather, was a rich industrialist, who owned a large number of wheat mills, and a fleet of ships that carried the wheat up and down the Volga, sailing under the Bashkiroff green-and-gold family flag.

Both grandfathers were as adventurous with women as they were with their investments. Pavel, a Cossack, was a widower in his fifties when he married a nineteen-year old peasant girl, Pelagia, who was working on one of his estates. Pelagia was a stunning beauty, spirited, and willing to spend hours with tutors—in "My Fair Lady" style—so she could be transformed into a cultured lady. Pavel fathered his last child with Pelagia at age seventy-five.

Nicholas Bashkiroff had ten children by his first wife, and then ran off with the wife of a captain of one of his ships, remarried and started a second family. Feodor, Sasha's father, was a son from the first marriage.

Feodor was encouraged to participate in the family business, although Sasha remembered his father as having little interest in serious matters.

"He'd go off to sell the wheat, only to return days later without the money because he had already spent it in another town having a good time," Sasha would recall disdainfully.

Sasha idolized his mother, Katya, born from Pavel and Pelagia's marriage, but he didn't have much respect for his father. "On one occasion my father took one of our family ships down the Volga and we never saw the ship again. My father claims he lost it. How do you lose a ship? He probably sold it to entertain his latest paramour."

Feodor's reputation as a roaming dilettante caught the fancy of a cartoonist who published a caricature of him in the Samara newspaper showing Feodor in the gray cape and the gray top hat that he always wore, captioned to paraphrase Pushkin: "What mysterious force drives you?"

Early in Sasha's childhood, his mother divorced his father. Their marriage had produced three sons, Gyorgy, Boris, and Sasha, with Sasha being the youngest. The three boys were raised from birth by maids and governesses, and Sasha's boyhood memories of his mother were mainly limited to an ethereal vision in ermine, jewels, and lingering perfume who used to brush by his bedroom to kiss him goodnight before going off to a ball.

As a child, the only memory of his father showing him any affection was one awkward gesture. It took place in a bathroom when his father came into the room, watched for a moment, and then patted him approvingly on the head and said, "Pee well and I'll buy you a pony."

Sasha's family owned so many estates that no one had ever visited them all. Italian and French architects were brought in to design their mansions, and botanists were hired from Moscow to cultivate lavish formal gardens and their own private orchards.

Sasha's Aunt Shura was given property as a birthday present, and it was on this land that Maxim Gorki wrote one of his stories. Sergei Prokofiev, the composer and pianist, used to attend musical evenings at the St. Petersburg home of the poet Boris Verin (pen name) Bashkiroff, Sasha's half-uncle. Verin and his brother, Vladimir Bashkiroff, were close friends of Prokofiev and years later assisted him financially when he lived in Europe.

For the rich the era before the Revolution was a time of overindulgence. One of Sasha's relatives resided in Cannes, France, most of his life, but he missed the fresh sturgeon—the sterlet—from Russia. This was remedied by the hiring of a manservant whose only duty was to travel back and forth by train, between Russia and France, escorting the sturgeon. Another relative, Sasha's Uncle Volodia, often ordered fresh violets to be delivered to him in Samara in the middle of the winter. A bachelor who enjoyed the art of wooing women, Volodia had the violets braided into his horse's mane to impress his lady friends.

Sasha was particularly fond of his Uncle Volodia. On sunny spring days before the snow melted, Volodia would take Sasha on sleigh rides across the meadows and they'd stop and listen to the sound of thawing ice cracking like distant thunder on the Volga. Sometimes, as a special treat, he'd allow Sasha to hold the reins of the horses.

When Sasha became a teenager his Uncle Volodia introduced him to pickle juice as a cure for a hangover. A German governess, Fraulein Mueller, was responsible for the more serious lessons in Sasha's life. Fraulein Mueller taught Sasha to speak German fluently, and to line up his shoes when he took them off, toe to toe. Her lessons in exactness and fastidiousness became so much a part of Sasha's character that even as an adult he lived as if Fraulein Mueller were looking over his shoulder. Yet he adored his governess.

And as a teenager he also soon discovered the sweetness of romantic love. Sasha's mother usually hired young Latvian maids because they had a reputation for cleanliness and hard work. Sasha had just turned fourteen years old when he came across his brother Gyorgy huddled with one of the maids in the darkness of the long hallway leading to the bedrooms. He saw Gyorgy nestle his face in the girl's neck, and heard her soft laughter. For a long while afterwards, Sasha's reaction toward these maids was a mixture of shyness and sexual curiosity.

There was a maid who used to tease Sasha when they were alone. Sometimes she would ruffle his hair as she passed him, and at first Sasha acted offended, as young boys do at any sign of affection, but as time passed her touch became embarrassingly important to him.

One day she entered his room and without saying a word she took one of his hands, played with the fingers, and then lifted the hand and placed it against her breast. When Sasha pulled his hand away she took it again, and this time she opened the front of her dress and let his hand slide down until it touched a nipple.

It was their secret game, at first innocently contained to kisses and quick caresses. Finally, one night she came into his bed.

Sasha's family was Russian Orthodox, but they rarely attended church. Sasha was brought up with the belief that "God is in us wherever we are."

Although the family took advantage of all the privileges their wealth could buy, they were not blind to the widespread poverty among the Russian peasants. As the years went by they became more and more critical of the inequities of life under the tsarist regime. Indeed, an atmosphere of opposition to the regime developed among many educated and wealthy families.

When they went to their home in Moscow, Katya would walk miles to hear the revolutionaries. Sometimes she would take her sons Boris and Sasha with her. They would try to push their way toward the front of the crowd so they could get a closer view of the speakers. Red had become the symbolic color of the revolutionaries and to show her sympathy toward the demands for "land to the peasants, factories to the workers" Katya often wore a red carnation pinned next to her jewels.

It was a relative who warned them, "It's all very well to listen to these speeches, but I can assure you if the revolutionaries win, you'll live to regret it."

His prophecy came true too soon. Toward the end of 1918, Sasha's brother Boris became a volunteer in the White Army. He joined not because he particularly wanted to fight the Bolsheviks, but because he was young enough and naive enough to believe this was a way to leave home and "become a man." He soon discovered the reality of the Revolution.

On April 4, 1919, Boris wrote to Sasha:

> Although it is a bore to repeat what I have already written, still in short, I will describe my life in Siberia.
>
> After we parted in Ufa, I spent a month travelling in cattle cars. I arrived in Barnaul, from where I went to Tomsk just a month ago. In Barnaul, it could not have been worse. Cold—47 degrees C. Without clothes and boots; dressed in thin torn shoes; empty stomach, and on top of it all, I became ill. As soon as we got settled in this hole, I contracted terrible chills and fever. Then, from the dirt, I became covered with pus-infected boils, resulting in my having to have my left leg and hand lanced three separate times. This is how I spent Christmas: lying on bare boards, wrapped in torn, louse-infected chenille, shirt and longjohns in the same condition, which were the only ones I had. I howled so that the entire regiment heard me.
>
> Accidentally I found out that Uncle Volodia is at present in Tomsk, and as they are disbanding our regiment in Barnaul, I went to Tomsk, where I am at present.
>
> Here, thank God, they gave me military clothing so I cannot complain too much.
>
> Well, enough about myself. I am much more interested in all of you than in myself. I wanted to write to you for a long time, but you are to blame. You wrote to Uncle Volodia without giving a return address. I am concerned that this letter and the telegrams I have sent you may also get lost and not reach you.

At the same time Sasha received a letter from his Uncle Volodia who, despite the Revolution, still enjoyed a sumptuous style of living.

Wrote Volodia: "I just returned from the Dvoryansky Sobranya [Nobleman's Club], where I ate borscht, goulash, two
whipped-cream cakes and drank a glass of coffee. Became very
ill and was worried that I would kick the bucket, which I don't
want to do," he joked. His letter went on:

> I think we shall soon see each other because the news
> from the front lines is more comforting with each pass
> ing day. And, God willing, it will soon be that we will
> find ourselves back home. Unfortunately, however, we
> will no longer have the kind of carefree life we had in
> the past.
>
> I found a buyer, a local millionaire who has a candy
> factory, and sold my horses to him for 15,000 rubles. As
> a bonus I received half a sack of candy, which I
> "shoveled into myself" with great pleasure.
>
> One of the horses, "Intrigue," immediately got shipped
> to Krasnoyarsk, and "Defender" remained in Tomsk, and
> was resold to another owner for 7,000 rubles. The new
> owner will race her tomorrow. I, of course, will go to the
> races too, and will bet 10 rubles on her and probably
> win about 200 rubles, which will be very pleasant.
>
> A telegram has just been received regarding the capture
> of Ufa. The officer who brought this news to the mess
> hall was picked up bodily and thrown in the air. This
> conquest brings the possibility of the recapture of
> Samara, in which case we will soon return home.
>
> To tell you the truth, I am tired of living in cold
> Tomsk. You will be surprised that I changed writing
> from black ink to red—this is in celebration of the happy
> news.
>
> I kiss you and hope to see you soon.
>
> > Your uncle.

The last time Sasha saw his brother Boris was in Chelyabinsk, a town near the Ural Mountains where Boris was
stationed.

The visit was short, less than forty-eight hours. The brothers left the chaotic, makeshift army barracks, and the pensive faces of other teenage soldiers who had seen too much, and made their way into the countryside. There they sat on rocks and talked of their boyhood years in Samara, reminiscing like old men who prefer to dwell only on the good memories.

When it was time for Sasha to leave they headed toward the train station by cutting a path through a field of tall, golden wheat. The wheat rippled with the wind as they walked, its beauty a gentle refuge in a land being defaced by man-made ugliness.

"You must get back to your barracks now," urged Sasha. "You will get into trouble."

"I will walk with you a little further," said Boris.

After a while Sasha reminded him, "Now you must go," but Boris remained with Sasha, reluctant to leave him. At last they stopped. The two brothers embraced and Sasha stood and watched as Boris turned back into the field. While he walked Boris kept waving to Sasha, and even when the distance increased between them he continued to wave until Sasha could only see his hand above the wheat. Then Boris disappeared from Sasha's sight.

A few months later Boris caught typhus. At the same time his encampment was overrun by the Reds and he was captured. Neither the White nor the Red armies had the resources or the desire to care for sick prisoners. Boris was shot.

Gyorgy, Sasha's other brother, had left home years earlier, married young, and the family had lost track of him. After the Revolution started they feared that he, too, had been killed.

Meanwhile, Sasha was drafted into the Cossack regiment as a cavalryman. As part of their training, the young recruits were forced to ride bareback. When they complained that their thighs were raw from gripping the flanks of the horses, the camp doctor's remedy was to splash iodine against the smarting skin. The fierceness of the iodine was nothing compared to the Russian winter, which caught the cavalry unprepared in their summer uniforms. There were times when Sasha thought he would become one more frozen mound in the bleak white landscape.

As the Civil War intensified, Katya became concerned not only about Sasha's safety, but also her own. Their family estates in Samara were under control of the revolutionaries, and Katya was now living near the Ural Mountains. She wanted to move further away from the fighting but she refused to leave the area without Sasha.

Katya arranged a secret meeting with a high-ranking officer, and one evening when the moon gave off little light, this officer visited Sasha at his camp and quickly separated him from the other men. Then he put a cape around himself, an identical one around Sasha, and they locked arms and walked away from the camp, their staggering silhouettes implying they were two officers soaked full of vodka.

Katya waited for Sasha at the railroad station. Her plan was to take the Trans-Siberian train eastward to any place where the fighting wasn't as intense. She was part of the frightened mass that had begun to drift aimlessly across the face of the land. Katya and Sasha knew if the Civil War didn't end they would ultimately have no choice but to leave the country and flee to Manchuria.

The Trans-Siberian train, once a symbol of luxury with its bath car and reading room-cum-library, was in chaos. Class distinctions in passenger coaches had been abolished. The sick, the wounded, women, children, and soldiers were jammed into deplorably filthy third-class cars or freight wagons, ventilated by winter winds that didn't dispel the odor of human excrement. For those who embarked upon such a journey, medicines were nonexistent and food scarce.

The Czechs, who had joined in the struggle against the Bolsheviks, now patrolled the Trans-Siberian. Katya took one Czech guard aside and gave him a hefty bribe to smuggle Sasha onto the already overcrowded cattle car. She could only hope the bribe would guarantee Sasha's safety, for Katya knew Sasha would be shot on the spot if it was discovered he had deserted his regiment.

For several days Sasha remained hunched in the cattle car, separated from Katya, who had managed to wedge her way into another section of the train with her maid. Hidden under Katya's clothing between her breasts and around her waist were soft silk bags containing some of her most precious jewels; to Katya these jewels had become her lifeline because vendors now had no faith in paper rubles and would only accept coins or articles of unquestionable value.

As the train journey progressed eastward, Sasha's knee began to swell from an injury he had received while in the cavalry. He became feverish and in his sleep he moaned loudly. During one of the train's stops the Czech guard, who had been bribed to look after Sasha, suddenly heard his moans and grew alarmed. He grabbed Sasha and forcibly pushed him out of the cattle car.

At that moment Katya and her maid were trying to squeeze their way along the platform to buy a chunk of bread from a vendor who was being besieged by the ravenous mob from the train. It was a matter of luck that Katya happened to be near enough the cattle car to spot Sasha being tossed out like a rag doll onto the ground. Katya immediately rushed to help her son, but the Czech guard caught her arm. He pulled her out of earshot of the other guards. "Your son is delirious," he explained angrily. "It's too dangerous for me to let him stay on the train anymore."

The train moved on, leaving Katya and Sasha stranded in the village. Katya's maid, afraid for her own life, stayed on the train, her loyalty to the family broken by the Revolution.

The snow veiled the countryside around them, and for a few minutes Katya stood with Sasha on the platform not knowing what to do. At last, with Sasha leaning on her arm they began to walk toward the village. As they approached the first log cabins they saw a child watching them.

"Please help us," Katya called out. "My son is hurt."

The child hesitated. Katya took out a coin and the youngster volunteered a smile and led them to his cabin. His parents were farmers, unsympathetic toward both the Reds and the Whites, but they took Katya and Sasha into their home, which consisted of only a single smoke-blackened room dominated by a massive masonry heating stove.

For two weeks Sasha and Katya slept in their barn, and during the day the peasant woman took large leaves, cooked them slowly, and then while they were still hot and steaming she pressed them against Sasha's injured knee, telling him these leaves would cure him. Little by little the swelling went down.

Sasha and Katya finally managed to bribe their way back onto the Trans-Siberian train and escaped to Manchuria, which had become a haven for White Russians.

They settled in Harbin and over the years Katya sold the jewels she had brought out from Russia. With this money she gave Sasha a good education, and he graduated from the Polytechnic Institute in Harbin with degrees in electrical and mechanical engineering.

Unlike his father, Sasha needed to get a job in a world that had totally changed from the one he was born into.

My maternal grandmother, Sophie, was born in Siberia, the land of the split personality; there is the Siberia known for its exiles and prison camps, and then there is the Siberia of silent majesty with its immense forests, steppes, mountains, and lakes. The people raised on this land, it is said, are *krepky narod*—strong people.

Sophie was the oldest daughter of twelve children, and the favorite child of my great-grandfather. When she was seventeen years old, Sophie fell in love with a soldier, Judah Rubinstein, who was stationed for a short time in Stretynsk, Sophie's hometown.

Both Sophie and Judah were Jewish, but Judah had been raised in the Ukraine, where Jews were persecuted. In the 1890s, Russian Jews could not always live where they liked, and the majority of Jews were legally restricted to ghettos within the so-called Pale of Settlement in western and south-western provinces of Russia. Judah was under strict orders to return to the Ukraine after completion of his military service.

In contrast, Jewish families in Siberia had escaped such religious oppression. Siberia had always been freer than European Russia. Due to the freethinking political exiles who were sent to the area, as well as the need to withstand the challenge of this rigorous land, the Siberians had developed a heritage of independence.

Sophie's father was head of the Jewish synagogue in Stretynsk and he had even traveled to Switzerland as the Siberian representative to an international Jewish congress, a journey which was a notable endeavor in the 1800s. He owned several stores, a soap factory, and six river passenger boats, gaining such importance as a businessman that he had been made a merchant of the first guild, a status that allowed him more privileges than most Jewish people. It was not surprising, therefore, that when Judah asked for permission to marry Sophie and take her back with him to the Ukraine, my great-grandfather refused to allow the marriage to take place; he didn't want his daughter moving thousands of miles away from him, to an area where she would be subjected to anti-Semitism.

However, just before Judah left Siberia, Sophie developed typhoid. To coax her back to health her father softened his position against the marriage and told her he would allow the wedding to take place as long as Judah found a way to remain in Siberia. With the help of my great-grandfather it was arranged for the couple "to disappear" after their marriage. Judah and Sophie went into hiding in the Siberian taiga, a vast coniferous forest where the trees grow so closely together they seem to swallow humans, a place for Judah to drop from sight until the authorities stopped looking for him.

They lived in one of the small, crude settlements that had been eked out of the taiga. Judah worked as a bookkeeper for a gold mine, and Sophie sewed shirts for the men, using wheat-flour bags as material. On July 26, 1895, nine months after their marriage, Aida, my mother was born.

Aida was a sickly baby, too frail to endure the harsh conditions of the forest. Sophie was forced to take her baby out of the taiga and leave her with her parents, hoping that under their care she would survive. It was an excruciating decision for her: a choice between leaving her husband or leaving her child. She chose to return to Judah in the taiga and didn't see her little girl for another year.

Eventually, Judah came out of hiding and he, Sophie, and Aida settled in Nikolaievsk, an important trading center located in the northernmost part of inhabited Siberia, at the mouth of the river Amur. Judah became a prominent businessman in Nikolaievsk, owning both fisheries and lumberyards. He and Sophie had three more children, and during all the years they lived together they remained devoted to one another; their marriage was one of our family's successful love stories.

When World War I was declared, Aida was in Germany studying piano at the Music Conservatory of Berlin. Recognizing that she would be considered an "enemy" because she was Russian, Aida left Germany immediately. On the long train journey back to Nikolaievsk my mother met a soldier named Yourieff. By the time the train reached Siberia, the two were talking marriage.

At first their courtship was limited to letters since Yourieff was in the army. In one letter Yourieff wrote about a love affair between another soldier and a married woman, describing how the married woman's husband discovered the pair, prompting the soldier to jump out of a window to escape the husband's wrath.

After Yourieff and Aida were married, Yourieff happened to repeat this story one night while they were in bed. He must have slipped on the details because all at once Aida's body stiffened as she lay next to him.

"You told me it was another soldier," she said. "It was you, wasn't it?" Then the tears came.

"Darling, we were not married at the time," protested Yourieff. "I am a man. It meant nothing to me."

My mother could be excessively jealous, and she lay there sobbing with such intensity that Yourieff—who also knew how to overplay the emotions—swung out of bed, fetched his revolver, and handed it to Aida.

"All right, here is my revolver. Shoot me," he challenged her.

Yourieff's death came a short time later, but not by Aida's hand.

Yourieff and Aida had made their home in Nikolaievsk to be near Judah and Sophie. Nikolaievsk-on-Amur was famous not only for its salmon fisheries and lumber, but also for its gold and fur exports. The town had no railroad connection, and although Nikolaievsk was a deep-water port, it was only accessible to large ships in the summer months. During the long Siberian winter, Nikolaievsk was cut off from the rest of the world, except for horse and dog sleighs, which carried fur-wrapped passengers along narrow snow-packed paths on the frozen river.

Toward the end of 1919, the population was about fifteen thousand, including approximately one thousand Kolchak White Guard soldiers and several hundred Japanese troops.

Siberia, by this time, was embroiled in grim battles, and pillaging. Guerilla organizations composed of revolutionary peasants and brigands raided the countryside. The Red Army had been stretched thin in Siberia, and the Soviets, in their effort to conquer this expansive land, relied on these partisan gangs for guerilla type war.

A young partisan leader, Yakov Triapitzin, was inhumanly brutal. Stories of his savage deeds had spread throughout Siberia. It was said that soldiers of the White Guard who fell into his hands often committed suicide, rather than be subjected to his torture. Triapitzin's lover, Nina Lebedeva, the second in command of his troops, was described as equally sadistic.

Yakov Triapitzin chose wintertime, February, 1920, when Nikolaievsk was set in frozen isolation from its neighbors, to attack the town. He and his followers had taken control of a fortress near Nikolaievsk that had several cannons, and his men threatened to bombard Nikolaievsk with these long-range guns if the Japanese troops who were stationed in Nikolaievsk didn't stop their support of the White Guards. The Japanese, armed with only rifles and machine guns, were no match for this threat and after a couple of days of negotiations they signed an agreement with Triapitzin.

As soon as Triapitzin's troops entered Nikolaievsk they arrested and killed all the White Guards. They even attacked the military hospital, pulled the sick White officers out of their beds, and beat them to death in front of the nurses. They then raped the nurses and threw them into prison.

Triapitzin's men searched every house in Nikolaievsk looking for bourgeois. Judah and Sophie were away in Europe, but Yourieff and Aida knew their lives were in danger, especially since Yourieff had served in the White Army. They had just had a baby, a girl called Berta (Betty), and Aida bundled her child in several layers of clothing and sought refuge at friends' homes. She had to move frequently because even life-long friends were afraid to harbor them for fear of reprisal.

Yourieff decided to seek asylum in one of the town's consulates. He selected the Japanese consulate. It was the wrong move. The Japanese garrison and the Japanese consulate still presented a threat to Triapitzin, so the partisans attacked the Japanese consulate killing everyone, including Yourieff. Eventually they slaughtered the entire Japanese population.

It became a blood bath. Triapitzin and his men systematically massacred thousands of Russians. Almost every household in Nikolaievsk lost some member, and a number of my relatives were killed. Even women and children were shot or bayonetted. Some people were pushed alive into holes dug in the frozen Amur river.

My grandparents and the Lury family, my grandfather's sister and brother-in-law, owned large homes in Nikolaievsk, and these were occupied by Triapitzin and his troops. In one of the rooms of my grandparents' house there was an old safe, and when Triapitzin saw it, he ordered his men to search Nikolaievsk for my mother so she could open the safe for him.

They found Aida and dragged her back to her father's home. "Open it!" Triapitzin's men demanded, pushing her toward the safe.

"The lock is broken. I swear it!" pleaded Aida. "My family hasn't used the safe for years." Her hand shook.

"Open it," they repeated, and one man took his rifle and held it at her throat. "I beg you," she implored, as she tried to juggle the lock, "my father told me this lock is jammed. I doubt if there is anything in the safe."

Unexpectedly, as Aida continued to frantically twist the lock, the door of the safe swung open revealing a few papers on the shelves. Aida became even more petrified, not knowing whether the papers were politically sensitive, but the men glanced at the documents, dismissed them as worthless, and threw them on the floor. Now Triapitzin's men turned their full attention on Aida. They lashed out insults labeling her a bourgeois, a leech, a parasite of the poor.

Ironically, Aida had always been the liberal in the family. Even as a young child she had upset family gatherings by criticising her parents for not sharing their money with the poor. As the men continued to insult her, she became righteously indignant, anger suddenly quelling her fear.

"I'm not a parasite," she retorted, facing them boldly. "I am a piano teacher. I give lessons, so I am a useful member of society."

Her lofty defense of herself amused Triapitzin's men. Said one crudely, "If you're such a good pianist, why don't you play us a love song?"

Aida walked over to her father's piano, sat down, and played romantic songs to cutthroats who laughed at her and then let her go with the warning that they might call on her again.

Aida finally managed to escape with her baby to a Chinese gunboat that was anchored on the Amur for the winter. They stayed on the boat until spring when the Japanese relief forces arrived in Nikolaievsk. These Japanese soldiers found the town destroyed, burned to the ground by Triapitzin's men, who had run off into the taiga.

After the Nikolaievsk massacre Aida went to live in Tsingtao, one of China's most popular coastal resorts, located on the Shantung Penisula where the beaches were wide and warm, with the grandeur of the Loashan Mountain as a backdrop. There my mother recuperated enough to fall in love again.

Solomon Bernstam was also a Siberian. He had the looks and the charm to attract many women, and was engaged when he met Aida. He swiftly broke off the engagement and married Aida instead.

It was not a happy marriage. In many ways Aida and Solomon were an unlikely pair. Aida was well educated, but Solomon had been drafted into the White Army at an early age and consequently had received little schooling. His speech was punctuated with Siberian idiom, which Aida corrected for the rest of their married lives.

The Nikolaievsk massacre traumatized Aida to such an extent that afterwards she lived in a constant state of apprehension. She became overly cautious, all her actions subjected to, "What if . . . ?" Solomon, on the other hand, was a risk-taker, his philosopy being, "Why not? Why worry? Tomorrow will take care of itself."

Early in their marriage Aida appeared to be on the edge of a nervous breakdown. Her doctor advised her, "You should have another child. It will settle your nerves."

And so I was born.

I was an anxious, imaginative child, prone to sleepwalking and daydreaming. Neither parent had the time nor the nature to nurture such a child. My father had difficulty showing affection, and my mother had difficulty coping with anything beyond her own problems. Aida never got over the tragedy of her first marriage, and the financial and emotional problems of her second marriage induced real and imaginary illnesses. There were times when she stayed in bed for days on end.

From birth I was left in almost total care of my Chinese amah. My grandparents, Judah and Sophie, were dismayed to find when they visited Tsingtao around my fifth birthday that they couldn't understand me because I only spoke Chinese.

My father was a skillful poker player, and every month he held poker parties for his men friends at our house. Our manservant, Tung, was fascinated with my father's imperturbability. Once, after the departure of the guests, Tung came to my mother and said, "Missy, all the men good—but our master best. Never move one eye."

Father's approach to life reflected this skill, and he was respected by the international business community in Tsingtao. One of my father's better ideas was the development of a racecourse in Tsingtao, which became well known, and for years we kept about ten Mongolian ponies. However, although he had a flair for putting together business deals, he was not always careful with business details. He'd enrich others, but he only occasionally benefited from these deals himself. Practically all his life my father teetered between financial highs and lows, which made my already nervous mother even more nervous.

While I was growing up I found my mother distant and almost forbidding. It wasn't until I became an adult that I understood the hardships my mother had faced, and appreciated her for the extraordinary woman she was.

Aida, who had once wanted to be an actress, tended to overdramatize most situations in life. My father's devil-may-care attitude, along with his numerous affairs, only fueled her histrionics. I remember seeing my mother, upon discovering my father was having another affair and even thinking of divorce, fainting with theatrical timing in our dining room while we were all watching her.

Although the Nikolaievsk massacre happened before I was born, Triapitzin emerged as the monster of my childhood. He was dangled before me threateningly. If I was bothered about some problem, my mother would say, "What do you have to cry about? You should have lived through Triapitzin."

There was no way I could compete with Triapitzin.

Due to my father's business ventures, we were constantly traveling between China and Japan. I learned to adapt to a kaleidoscopic view of the world, which proved beneficial, but the jumps from one country to another, from school to school, gave my upbringing little stability.

Although I was Jewish, the first school I attended was Catholic, the Convent of the Holy Ghost. Many Jewish girls were enrolled at this school because it offered an excellent education. I was a good student and won many prizes and awards, but both the nuns and my family also believed in teaching humility.

During a school award-winning ceremony, after my name had been mentioned several times, my grandfather turned to me and said, "You should not win everything. Give the other little girls a chance." He meant it as a joke. I took him seriously and cried on a day when I should have been happy.

It was a different story if one failed. A failure was something to dwell upon, to complain about forever. Or at least so it seemed. My sister, Betty, was the one who excelled in art, a subject I didn't like. The first time I got a low grade in drawing, my mother let it be known she was disappointed I wasn't as good as her older daughter.

"Mama, isn't it enough you have one artist in the family," I rationalized. "Why do you need two?"

I went through the English school system in the Orient, but because of the large number of consulates and international businesses in China, these schools were filled with students from many different countries. The teachers, as a matter of course, would begin a new year by asking each girl to stand up and identify her nationality.

By now, I had learned several languages including Russian. My parents had told me a little bit about their lives in Russia but, nevertheless, Russia to me was still an enigma. I was always conscious we had become stateless refugees.

When it came my turn to reveal my nationality I would reply, almost shamefully, "White Russian." It meant nothing. Except it meant a lot.

I was only fifteen years old when I first met Sasha. We were living in Shanghai, and our home was in the French Concession opposite Grosvenor House, a luxurious apartment complex where Sasha lived and worked.

Sasha had moved to Shanghai when he was in his thirties, and had obtained a prestigious job managing the properties of the multimillionaire Sir Victor Sassoon. The wealthy and the famous stayed in Grosvenor House, and Sasha had a large staff of masons, carpenters, and other technical experts who kept the building in top condition.

My bedroom looked onto the Grosvenor House gardens where nannies walked their starched-clothed children. The Grosvenor grounds were supposed to be used only by the tenants, but one day, ignoring the keep-out signs, I took a stroll through the gardens.

I hadn't gone very far before Sasha came up to me and inquired, "Excuse me miss, do you live here?"

I could tell by the way he looked at me that he already knew I didn't. I replied cheekily, "Yes, I do."

I had just started to be interested in the male sex, and to me Sasha was as handsome as any film star I had ever seen. I was dressed in custom-made shorts, white top, and saddle shoes. I thought I was grown-up. Then I saw the laughter on Sasha's face and I knew he still considered me a child. My fragile feelings of self-worth were hurt.

During the next five years I often heard people talk about Sasha, but whenever his name was mentioned I would say, scornfully, "Oh that pill!"

Chapter 2

FOR BETTER

When I was seventeen years old, I woke up one morning to find Shanghai occupied by the Japanese. The Second World War had arrived. The Japanese soldiers didn't say a word to us as we walked by them in the streets, their faces as inflexible as the barricades they had put up overnight to stop the flow of traffic.

Yet the next day the tension relaxed, most of the barricades were pushed aside, and it was back to business as usual. Shanghai was an international settlement that had learned its own survival techniques.

People became traders, buying and selling in a flourishing black market. Bolts of wool were swapped for flour, and in the end your own merchandise made its way back to you, ten times higher than the original price. One of the commodities my father traded was saccharine, and I remember sleeping with crates of saccharine hidden under the bed.

The rich and the very rich still went to their cabarets and restaurants, while the very poor begged, as they had always done, on the Shanghai streets. I used to walk by a Chinese beggar whose permanent place, except for late at night when the gang he belonged to picked him up, was on the sidewalk around the corner from my home. He was a quadriplegic who attracted the attention of the people on the street by bouncing his torso in front of them, juggling the tin that was chained to his handless arm. Every day I put coppers in the tin.

The Japanese took over many of the apartment houses for their military personnel. Our family, like many other families, was forced to leave our home and move in with relatives. When apartments became scarce, the middle and upper-income people invented a real-life Monopoly game using "key-money." A price was placed upon apartment keys, a figure that could be in the thousands. People sold these keys—even if they didn't own the apartment—and desperate families who had to have a place to live bought them, knowing they could still be evacuated by the Japanese.

As the European refugees began to descend upon Shanghai, my parents offered their help. Our home became an open door for destitute refugees in need of food or shelter. My mother also contracted a restaurant to provide a free daily lunch to the German and Austrian Jewish refugees; she persuaded her friends and the business people in the Russian Jewish community to pay for these lunches, and my mother and I often served as volunteer waitresses in the restaurant. After the war, my mother received a certificate from the Jewish refugees, honoring her for the help she gave them.

We were also aware of the atrocious crimes being committed against the Jews in Germany. Because we were stateless Russians we were comparatively safe in Shanghai but we had relatives who had lived abroad and had acquired American and British passports, and they were placed in concentration camps. The plight of others was an abscess on our minds, but wartime has a way of teaching you to block out the horrors and live only for the present. War even generates a certain excitement; lives speed up as people charge into each day, doing all the things they might not have done if there hadn't been a doubt about tomorrow.

It was in this atmosphere I began dating, fell in love with a man called Sandor, and lost my virginity. I didn't meet Sasha again until I was twenty years old, and by that time my relationship with Sandor had ended, the war showed no signs of ending, and I was only a little bit wiser about the ways of the world and men.

I ran into Sasha at a party. We talked about a book dealing with the state of the economy. I acted knowledgeable about the book, and he acted interested in me. Neither of us mentioned that years ago he had chased me out of the Grosvenor Gardens.

A couple of days after the party, Sasha saw me riding my bicycle near my home and called out, "Hello beautiful." It didn't take long before he invited me to have dinner with him.

At first it seemed odd for me to be with a man who was twenty years my senior. Many times I told myself: This is not right. I should be dating someone my age. Yet other times I mused: I wonder if I could make an older man fall in love with me? It was a playful thought, from a young woman with a childlike view of life as a game.

Ironically, I was the first one to realize I was in love. The years between us didn't appear to matter, and neither did the fact he wasn't Jewish. The difference in our religion was never even mentioned, perhaps because we were both nonconformists; I didn't go to temple and Sasha didn't go to church.

It was Sasha's complex personality that began to intrigue and enchant me. A great deal of Sasha's charm was that he seemed unaware of how handsome he was. Dark-complected, he had hazel eyes, an elegant straight nose, and a smile that gave the impression of introspection and wisdom. There was also a tenseness about him, a sense of withheld energy. He was not that tall, five feet eleven, but his training as a gymnast when he was young had given him a good posture and a powerful physique. Usually he dressed conservatively in tweed jackets, flannel pants, and bow ties.

His refined heritage was an implicit part of his character, and to those who did not know him well he could convey the effect of being haughty, when in reality he was an unpretentious and gentle man. For instance, when gasoline became scarce in Shanghai during the war, and practically the only way to get around effortlessly was in a rickshaw pulled by a coolie, Sasha refused to sit in these rickshaws, preferring to ride his own bicycle, or walk. He couldn't stand the thought of another human being carrying him.

Sasha readily expressed sentiment and emotion. He was the consummate gentleman, a creation of old-world courtliness who greeted all women with a suave kiss on the hand, and yet he was also capable, especially when he had had a few drinks, of layering the charm with a certain Cossack wildness. Once during a heated political argument at an Easter party in Shanghai, Sasha thrust his fist into the kulich, a Russian Easter cake, which had taken the hostess hours to make.

Before World War II, Sasha mixed socially with many of his tenants at Grosvenor House, including Leighton Shields, the U.S. Attorney to China at that time. It was Leighton Shields, the American, who taught Sasha Bashkiroff, the Russian, how to drink scotch by the fifth. When the war started and the Japanese took over the occupancy of Grosvenor House, Leighton was one of the few American tenants who was temporarily allowed to remain in the building, due to wartime diplomatic immunity.

One evening when Sasha was with Leighton in his apartment drinking, the talk turned to the United States. Suddenly Sasha opened a window, stuck his head out, and in a voice loaded with scotch and passion, sang "God Bless America." Sasha knew all the words. The Japanese officers who were living in Grosvenor House must have heard Sasha, but fortunately chose to ignore him. He could have been sent to prison for this act of singing a nationalistic song of the enemy.

Another time Sasha decided to practice his gymnastic skills—also under the influence of alcohol—in Leighton's apartment, and before Leighton could stop him Sasha climbed outside the apartment window, and hung by his hands, bending his body into pretzel maneuvers, twelve stories above the ground. Leighton, horrified, urgently called for his household help who carefully pulled Sasha back into the apartment.

These stories about Sasha enlivened the Shanghai gossip circuit, as did the stories of his past in Russia. The more I got to know Sasha, the more he would tell me about his family, detailing the richness of their lives not only in monetary terms, but in their culture. He spent hours describing what it meant for him to be Russian. Until I met Sasha I had no sense of nationality, but as I listened to Sasha I felt, for the first time, some pride in my own history.

Our favorite song was "You Belong To My Heart," and whenever there was a dance, Sasha would ask the band to play that number. We often visited the Bubbling Well Road cemetery, a place so full of elaborate statues that it resembled an art gallery. By the silent stone angels and carved-out poems we would stop and kiss.

For a long time we weren't sexually intimate, partly because Sasha thought I was still a virgin, but mainly because he felt it wasn't right for us to be intimate since he had no marriage plans. In many ways he was modern, but in this way he was old-fashioned. Sasha had been married once, and although the marriage had lasted ten years he rarely talked about the relationship. He would only tell me that he wasn't good husband material, and had no intention of remarrying, or having children.

I believe he also feared making an emotional commitment in a wartime climate. He was a man without a country who knew once the war ended he would probably have to move on. He didn't know where. That was the foremost thought on the minds of many people: If the Communists claimed Shanghai where could they go? The decisions people had to make in those days were difficult. Many made reckless decisions. Sasha moved cautiously.

Marriage, or any type of permanent relationship, wasn't on my mind either. I was still testing life and enjoying my independence.

I had been employed as a secretary in a large British department store before the war started. From the department store I went into teaching, and for three years I taught at the Jewish school I had attended as a child. I loved the work, and also used to tutor privately.

One of my private students was a young German girl. It was mandatory for Germans to send their children to the German school in Shanghai, but these parents didn't want their child subjected to the Nazi indoctrination being practiced at the school so they kept her at home, using the excuse the girl was sick.

Although I knew this family was anti-Nazi it still shocked me to find when I entered their home one morning a portrait of Hitler in their hallway. As a Jew I was tempted to leave and never return to their home but wartime had also taught me not to take things at face value. This family, I realized, hung Hitler's portrait purely because the father worked for a German company and had to show, at least outwardly, support for the Nazis. Either that or he would have lost his job.

So we both kept our jobs. I stayed on as the tutor, learning compassion for a family that was forced to live a lie, teaching compassion to a child who wanted to grow up without Hitler's propaganda.

The war was over. We heard rumors the Americans would soon occupy Shanghai but we didn't know when. Then, one night, I attended a party at a friend's house and as I walked into the living room I was amazed to see several Americans standing there in full military uniform.

My friend, Igor, had pulled off a scoop. He had heard over the shortwave broadcasts that there were Japanese surrender planes, marked with crosses, at the Shanghai airport. Igor was one of the few people in Shanghai who still had a car, although he didn't have a permit to drive it. Regardless, he got into his big Chrysler and drove out to the airport.

Igor arrived just in time to see ten American military men stepping off a plane, the first American military mission to land in Shanghai. The men immediately spotted Igor and his Chrysler.

"Hi, can you give us a ride into the city?" yelled one of the Americans to Igor. To Igor, this casual, friendly greeting was a graphic sign that the Americans had indeed arrived. Shanghai was very British in demeanor—reserved and polite in official matters—and this cheerful casualness of strangers piling into his car could have only happened with Americans!

On their way into the city, Igor decided to throw a victory party in honor of the conquering heroes. He kept the presence of the Americans a secret from his guests when he extended the invitations; it was the best surprise party we had ever attended. It took two servants to carry the commemorative cake to the table—an elaborate creation baked in the shape of an American flag.

As soon as the Japanese surrender was official, the American military personnel moved into the Park Hotel in Shanghai, next to the YMCA, which was still occupied by the Japanese High Command. The two sides, adhering to military protocol, used to salute each other as they went in and out of the buildings.

For months after the Japanese surrender we celebrated, letting go of all the tension and fear that lock inside of you during a war. Shanghai became the port of departure to the United States, so every day more and more American military men arrived in Shanghai to be processed and sent on their way home. All at once there were too many men around, and too many parties. For a short time we erased the past, didn't think about the future, and acted outrageously.

It was then Sasha realized that if our relationship didn't become more intimate he might lose me to the American officers, who were more than willing to court me, make love to me, marry me, anything. American soldiers were handing out marriage proposals as generously as they handed out their cigarettes.

I wasn't a beauty although people told me I was attractive. I was fortunate enough to be slim with a good figure, except I would have liked to have had a flatter behind. When I was a young woman I was never quite satisfied with my appearance. As a child I had blond hair, but as I got older I had become a brunette. With a little help from a hairdresser I had turned into a blond again and I kept my hair short and stylish.

Said one of my friends, "Anne, it's up to you. With your good looks you could marry an admiral, a general, whoever you want."

Said Sasha, "When you are coming to stay overnight with me?"

To Sasha I kept replying, "Tomorrow"—meaning, after all this time of knowing him the idea of sex with him scared me. Also, with the American officers in town I wasn't so sure I wanted to be tied just to Sasha.

Eventually Sasha said, somewhat seriously, "Either you come and stay with me tonight, or we'll call the whole thing off."

It was arranged. I lied to my parents, telling them I was going to stay with a girlfriend. Early in the evening I went to a party, and it was late when I walked into Sasha's apartment complex. Sasha was the only civilian now living in Grosvenor House; after the Japanese left, the American military personnel had taken over the building.

By the time I got to Sasha's door my slick attempt at sophistication had evaporated. After all, I was not what one might call "experienced." Sandor had been my only lover. The first time Sandor fondled me intimately we were in a courtyard

near my home in Shanghai. The night was dark enough for me
to think we were hidden in the shadows of the grass. As I lay on
the ground I wasn't sure what to do, or what he was doing.

Before Sandor, the only naked men I had seen were fishermen, when I was living in Japan at the age of twelve. The
fishermen used to stand unashamedly nude on the beach,
pulling in their nets. They would sing as they worked, words
monotonously repeated until the nets came closer, and then the
tempo of the song would speed up and become rhythmic. We
knew as the beat got faster that the fish were closer, and we
waited in anticipation for the net to free itself from the water,
overflowing with its shimmering, silver catch. As children we
would look at the fish, and slyly glance at the males' genitals,
and be fascinated by it all.

With Sandor I was still too young to do anything more than
merely glance at my man. And now with Sasha I was still too
nervous to enter into love-making without bashfulness. Sasha
came to the door in his dressing gown. I stood in the hallway
looking at him as if I didn't know him.

"Come on in," he urged, seeing my hesitation.

"I don't know if I am staying."

"Of course you're staying. Come on, take your coat off."

"No, I'm not going to take my coat off. I'm going to sit here,"
and I placed myself on a chair in his living room, my back to his
open bedroom door. I needed to be cajoled, to be told it was
okay.

Sasha put his arm around me, led me to the sofa and talked to
me.

In the morning Sasha took me on the back of his bicycle to
the school where I was teaching, and we agreed to meet again in
the afternoon. By four o'clock it was raining, but we went for a
walk in the rain, our heads together under one umbrella.

Sasha must have been concerned about what had happened

between us because he kept asking me, "Was I happy with him? Was I satisfied?"

I was embarrassed by his questions. In those days you didn't speak of sex the way you do today. He even asked if he had been all right. It astonished me that a man who had been married would want such reassurance from a young woman, and I didn't know how to respond.

"I'm very happy," I said simply. I meant it. I was in love and making love, and I couldn't wait to tell one my best friends, Trudi.

I had known Trudi since I was a teenager. Part French and part Austrian, Trudi had fled Hitler and moved to Shanghai. At first she came to my house to give me French lessons, but we soon met purely for friendship.

She had a kind, beautiful face and when Trudi listened and digested my life with me I always felt calmer. It was almost as though she were a soothsayer for me.

It was Trudi who told me over and over again that Sasha was the right man for me. "He has inner strength, inner resources," she used to say. "You need somebody as steady as this. Trust me. Pursue him."

I had invited Trudi to my twenty-second birthday party, an event that took place a few days after Sasha and I became lovers. As soon as Trudi arrived at the party I pulled her towards the bathroom. "I have something to tell you," I whispered. I locked the bathroom door so no one else could come in.

In that cramped space, with Trudi balanced on the edge of the bath, I told her, "Guess what? It happened. I stayed the night with Sasha."

"Anne, I'm thrilled for you," replied Trudi, hugging me. "Tell me all about it." Trudi had long ago advocated the seduction of Sasha.

I told her everything, how it happened, and what happened.

In some way, Trudi probably understood the significance of the sexual experience more than I did.

I continued to make love with Sasha whenever we met at his apartment. The apartment was sparsely furnished, for the Japanese had taken all of Sasha's furniture when they occupied the building. He had only been able to retrieve a few pieces, and none of the windows had drapes. When we made love Sasha used to cover the bedroom window with his raincoat.

It was Sasha who got me a job with the American Armed Forces. Although I had enjoyed teaching, the Americans lured many of us away from our jobs because it was considered more exciting to work for "the heroes." And then there was the promise of money. Lots of it. As soon as the Americans set up offices, they offered salaries many times higher than anything else you could get in Shanghai. Even the simplest clerk received a fantastic salary.

In retrospect, I consider their generosity in salaries unnecessary and disruptive to the Shanghai society, as well as a waste of the American taxpayers' money. Years later I became angry at the American system that could throw away money so readily to foreigners, and yet not give money to those people in their own country who really needed it.

However, while the Americans stayed in Shanghai we were intoxicated by our freedom. This freedom fogged our minds and it was only when the Americans began to withdraw that the political situation became far too clear. Realizing the inevitability of the Communists taking over Shanghai, we started to scurry about trying to obtain exit visas.

My sister, Betty, had emigrated to the United States before the war. Since Betty had become an American citizen my mother was given a top-priority immigration visa so she could join her daughter in the United States. I was not as lucky. I was told I might have to wait years to get a quota visa for America. The only other way for me to enter the United States was as a student.

With the help of my sister's husband, I applied to the University of California, Los Angeles, and was accepted.

Sasha was also trying to emigrate to the United States, but he didn't know what his chances were on the quota system.

My mother and I traveled to America together. Throughout her marriage my mother had always threatened to leave my father. Finally she did it. On the day we boarded the ship my mother walked out of her apartment, left her furniture, her dog, and her husband. Aida let my father know she was paying him back for all his infidelities. She walked away from him and all her belongings as casually as if she were going shopping.

Sasha came to see me off. We sat on the ship's deck, pressed together, and I cried until my face seemed as wet as the water around us.

I didn't think I would see him again.

A few days after I arrived in Los Angeles, I received a telegram from Sasha: "Will you marry me darling? Can't live without you. Love Sasha."

Six months later Sasha arrived in the United States. I met him at the dock and two hours after he got off the ship we were married.

Only a certain number of people were being allowed into the United States, but because of the increasing panic in Shanghai, Sasha had decided not to wait for his quota number to come up and had travelled to the United States on a transit visa. We hoped that somehow the authorities would let Sasha stay in America but to our dismay he was given ninety days to leave the country. Within those ninety days Sasha happened to receive his quota number, but despite our pleas that we now be given the legal right to remain in the country, the Immigration Department told us that since Sasha had switched to a transit visa, his quota number had become automatically invalid.

We were left with only one option. Sasha's brother Gyorgy, who the family thought had died in the Russian Revolution,

had turned up alive and living in Buenos Aires. Through
Gyorgy we managed to obtain a visa to Argentina. We stayed
there four years.

Buenos Aires, like Shanghai, was a night city. Even without
much money we were able to frequent clubs and cabarets,
lingering over full-course dinners at midnight. It was a glamorous start to a marriage, free of most responsibilities, with a
maid to clean our apartment, and a husband who was eager to
please me.

Sasha got a job as an engineer, and I found part-time
employment as a secretary to a patent attorney. One of the first
friends we made in Buenos Aires was a man of Russian
nobility, Nicholas Baranoff, who had lost his title of His Serene
Highness with the fall of the Russian Empire. Many years later
Nicholas became the godfather to our son.

Through Nicholas we met other high-ranking Russian families, including Basil Wyrouboff, whose aunt, Anna Vryubova,
had introduced Rasputin to the court of Nicholas and Alexan-
dra. A few of these Russian families had managed to get their
money out of Russia, but most of them escaped only with their
pride and memories. It was exciting for me to be included in
this sophisticated, multilingual circle of people, and once again
I felt I was discovering my own roots as I listened to them
describe their homeland and how much they missed it.

One evening we were invited to a dinner honoring the Grand
Duchess Marie of Russia, a cousin of Tsar Nicholas II. We were
a small party of eight, but it was a formal occasion and our host
and hostess followed established protocol, not allowing any of
the guests to drink until the Grand Duchess had arrived.

The Grand Duchess was thirty minutes late and I could see
that Sasha and some of the other men were getting impatient.
By the time Sasha was given permission to drink, he drank
quickly and heavily.

The sit-down dinner was at a rectangular table set with plates
of silver and gold cutlery. The ceilings in the house dripped

with crystal chandeliers, and every room was filled with Russian art, all probably brought out illegally.

During dinner, having had too much to drink, Sasha became quite boisterous and the hostess, who was sitting next to him, motioned to Sasha a couple of times, "Shh!"

Normally Sasha was conscious of good manners, but when he had had a few drinks I never knew what to expect. On this occasion he didn't give a damn about protocol and wanted to have fun, not sit at a prolonged, stiff dinner. He started to sing.

This time the hostess touched his hand, leaned over and whispered tersely, "Sasha, do you have to be so loud? The Grand Duchess is here."

It's important to understand that although Sasha loathed the communist system that had driven him out of Russia, he had also never forgotten that the Revolution was ignited by the arrogant refusal of the Tsar's regime to rectify Russia's unjust social conditions. Perhaps these thoughts were running through Sasha's mind when he slammed his fist down on the table and shouted, "To hell with the Grand Duchess. If it weren't for the Grand Duchess and her family I'd be back in my Samara."

I was, needless to say, mortified, but as time went on I learned to admire Sasha's forceful, and many-sided, personality.

His use of words was a colorful part of his character. He didn't learn the English language until he was in his thirties but his English was excellent, except he rolled his "r's" like a Frenchman. Otherwise, one might take him for an Englishman, sprinkling his sentences with "piffles" or "I beg your pardon," or "absolutely" pronounced vehemently, "ahbsolutely."

In the heat of an argument he adopted flamboyant rhetoric and liked nothing better than to use some curdling, descriptive Russian oath. I collected some choice phrases from Sasha. He'd often say about himself or his male friends—but never to me—"Ah ti, jopa galova" (Eh you, ass-head). Or if a room was in a mess, he'd utter, "*Nastoyashey bardak*" (Real whorehouse). Sasha always told me, "Don't be a *meschanka* (bourgeoise). Never be afraid of words."

I observed that all our Russian friends in Buenos Aires used obscene language freely. Sasha explained that in Russia it was perfectly acceptable for a gentleman to use such language because he obviously knew better, whereas if a less-educated person spoke in this way it would be offensive.

Sasha also had no hesitation about urinating outdoors, behind trees. He did it discreetly, usually when it was dark, a habit that probably went back to this country upbringing in Samara. Most of our friends in Buenos Aires understood this touch of eccentricity, although one friend, when we attended a party at her house, stressed to Sasha as he went out to use her garden, "Sasha darling, please use another tree. You have nearly killed my bougainvillaea."

In 1951 we were finally able to emigrate to the United States. It wasn't easy for us to settle in America because Sasha had difficulty finding work. At first we lived in Los Angeles and later moved to San Francisco; the newspapers in these cities were filled with engineering jobs but most of the firms were doing defense work and wouldn't hire Sasha since he wasn't a United States citizen.

As a result Sasha took any job that came along, saying to me, "I don't care what I do. I don't have to prove anything to anybody. I know who I am."

He had never worked as a physical laborer but he took a job building a corrugated roof, and I worked right beside him painting window trim. His willingness to attempt jobs where he wasn't particularly knowledgeable had a certain risk. When he became a sheet-metal laborer he dropped the sheet metal on his foot, and broke his toe. Another time while installing electrical wires on the mast of a ship for Bethlehem Steel, the coupling of a compressor hose hit Sasha on the inside of his eye, requiring stitches.

Then there was the time he applied for a job as a carpenter. Before he turned up for work at the construction company he went to a hardware store and asked the clerk, "What kind of tools would a carpenter need?"

The clerk sold Sasha an assortment of tools and put them in a cardboard box, tied up with string.

Sasha took the box of tools to work the next day and at noontime he felt great because he believed he had done a fine job.

Suddenly the foreman came up to him and said, "You're fired."

"Why?" asked Sasha, astonished.

"Because you're not a carpenter," said the foreman.

"How do you know I'm not a carpenter?" protested Sasha. "Look at what I did."

"No carpenter in the world would have come to work with new tools straight out of a box from the store," replied the foreman. That was the end of that job.

For one week Sasha found work as a draftsman, but they too fired him; Sasha had been away from drafting so long his skills had become rusty. He begged them to let him stay on, telling the boss he would work for nothing.

That night when Sasha came home and told me he had lost his drafting job he put his arms around me and cried. It was the only time I saw him discouraged.

Finally, Sasha was hired as an engineer for the American Can Company in San Francisco, and he stayed with this firm for eighteen years. I also found a job I loved as corporate secretary to Children's Hospital.

Shortly after my marriage to Sasha, my mother and father mended their marriage and they, too, ended up living in San Francisco. Sasha's own mother had died in Shanghai during

World War II, and I think Sasha welcomed the fact that my parents were living near us for he believed in strong family ties.

Yet he didn't want a child of his own. His experience in the Russian Revolution left a scar on Sasha; he would argue that life was too cruel and uncertain, and why should we bring such suffering upon an innocent child? After seven years of marriage when I found out I was pregnant, Sasha's response was an anguished, "How could you do this to me?"

Fortunately, with the birth of our son, Nicholas Alexander, his attitude about children completely changed. He revered his son, who was given Sasha's formal name of Alexander, and the name of Sasha's paternal grandfather, Nicholas Bashkiroff.

For years our marriage was a happy one. Often at night if Sasha heard a song he liked on the radio he would dim the lights, pull me out of my chair and we would dance, just the two of us, in our living room. As he held me close he would sometimes sing our song from Shanghai, "You Belong to My Heart." On other evenings we would play our Russian records, and Sasha would sing along with the records, echoing the fervent emotion that is an intrinsic part of this music. He had a true baritone voice, a wonderful gift which he could have developed professionally had the circumstances been different when he was younger. As a family we treasured his singing voice and music was very much part of our lives.

Eventually we became American citizens, bought our own house, and bought the American dream. We thought if we worked hard, had savings in the bank, and good insurance, and were good people, nothing could go wrong.

PART TWO

Chapter 3

FOR WORSE

It was Saturday, the day we did our grocery shopping. As soon as he finished breakfast Sasha began pushing me, "Come on, Anne, it's late. If we wait much longer the shops will be too crowded."

He appeared annoyed when the telephone rang and I started talking to a friend. Any minute I expected him to tell me, "Anne, get off the phone. Tell her you'll call her back."

Sasha thought nothing of interrupting my calls if he felt they were untimely. He would pace in front of me, ram me with unsubtle signals. On this morning, though, he gave me a cross look and left the room. When I hung up the telephone I called out to him I was ready to leave. I didn't get an answer. At first I suspected Sasha had become so impatient he'd gone shopping without me. I checked the garage. The car was there. I went back into the house and called his name again. There was still no reply.

I searched the rooms downstairs and then went upstairs. I found Sasha on our bed, his body wound into the fetal position. He was shivering violently.

"Honey, what's the matter?" I asked, bending over him. His face appeared greenish.

"I'm f-freezing." The words were squeezed out between the clattering of his teeth.

His shivering frightened me. I couldn't imagine what was wrong. We had been married twenty-two years and during all that time Sasha had rarely been sick.

Quickly, I pulled down some extra blankets from our cupboard, piled them on top of Sasha, and ran to wake Nicky who, like most fifteen-year-old boys, liked to sleep in whenever possible.

"Nicky, Papa isn't feeling well. Find some more blankets and try to keep him warm. I have to call the doctor."

Why do illnesses hit on weekends, when doctors are hard to reach? It took time to get the call through, but after hearing Sasha's symptoms our family physician didn't seem concerned.

"He's probably got the flu," he responded. "Does he have a fever?"

"He doesn't appear to have one."

"Is he throwing up?"

"No."

"Well, I'm sure it's the flu." The doctor sounded irritated I had bothered him. "Let me know if things change."

No sooner had I reached our bedroom door when I heard Sasha blurt out, "I'm going to be sick."

I managed to get a plastic wastebasket to him before he threw up.

I called the doctor back. His voice held the same sigh of: What now? You know this is Saturday.

The doctor's manner changed when I told him Sasha had vomited. "Okay, I'll be right over," he promised.

He was one of the few doctors who was still willing to come to a home. We had known him for a long time and were aware that his hobby was raising orchids, and even on this Saturday he arrived wearing a fresh orchid tucked in his lapel.

Nicky and I stood quietly by the bed while Sasha was examined. One of the doctor's first questions was whether Sasha had any pain in his back. Sasha motioned he did.

I was not prepared for the doctor's swift conclusion. "You have an acute kidney infection," he announced to Sasha. "You'll have to go to the hospital."

The doctor then placed a call to see if he could get a room, and while waiting for the hospital to call back, he and Nicky started to talk about photography, a hobby they both shared. Nicky gave the doctor his camera, and I watched as the doctor turned it over in his hands, fascinated by the camera's parts and possibilities.

I couldn't help but think how easy it was for a doctor to become detached from his patient's illness. One minute he could tell a man he has an acute kidney infection, and in the next minute stand near us, but mentally isolated from us, and toy with a camera.

I stood on the sidelines observing Nicky and the doctor talking, observing Sasha's head sunk into the pillow, while my own head reeled, as I tried to deal with the news Sasha was so ill.

The doctor drove us in his car to Children's Hospital, the same hospital where I worked. Shortly after we arrived, Sasha's temperature became hideously high and he lapsed into a coma.

He drifted in and out of consciousness for four days, the high temperature and infection raging within him. I was told he needed to have his kidney removed, but they couldn't operate until the fever subsided.

The doctors left me with the impression Sasha might die, although their words were carefully chosen, leaning on the phrase "very critical." Doctors have a way of avoiding the actual word "death."

I prayed.

And I panicked. We had enjoyed a traditional togetherness-type marriage. Sasha was always with me for he didn't have, or want, any interests that took him away from home. I wasn't used to being apart from him. Now, there was a stillness in the rooms, and at night my legs drifted too far across an empty bed. What if he should die?

I kept going to my job at the hospital for it was a way to keep my mind occupied. Besides, my office was near Sasha's hospital room. Every opportunity I had I visited him. If I thought Sasha looked worse I would track down the doctor and plead with him to do something.

The difficult part was in the evening when I was back in my house, not knowing if any change was taking place. I would call the doctor asking for a report until eventually the doctor became fed up with me.

"Take a sedative so you can go to sleep, but leave me alone," he scolded. "You can't keep calling me. I have to be awake in the morning to take care of your husband. You're not helping."

He didn't mean to be unkind. I knew I was being impossible but I was scared. The nurses, for the most part, dispensed platitudes, refusing to give out detailed information. I, on the other hand, rummaged for reassurance, for somebody to say something definite about my husband's condition. Was he getting worse? Better? Just tell me. Prepare me.

After the fourth day the fever finally broke, and the doctors told me they were ready to operate. On the morning of the surgery, I waited with Sasha until he was groggy, following him as he was wheeled down the hallway. When I couldn't go any further with Sasha, I went to my office.

I now felt empathy with faces I had seen in the hospital waiting rooms, faces that looked up anxiously when anybody neared them, mouths attempting normal conversation when nothing felt normal.

I watched the minutes pass on the office clock, my imagination entering the operating room. I saw it all, the mind's view worse than the real view. They had taken my husband away from me, and I was left to picture how they would bring him back.

One of the doctors I worked with realized I had driven myself into a terrible state. "I'll go down to the operating room if you like," he volunteered, "and see what's happening."

"Would you?"

"Sure." Off he went, my own sensitive spy.

He returned smiling. I sensed the relief before he even said anything. "It was successful, Anne. There were no complications. They removed the kidney and your husband tolerated it very well. You don't have to worry any more," he stressed soothingly. "It's all over and everything's going to be all right."

Immediately I telephoned Nicky at school.

Everything was going to be all right.

After the surgery I arranged to have Sasha placed in a private room. It didn't surprise me that on my first visit he didn't remember the operation for he looked and acted as if he were still submerged in anesthesia. But on the third day after the operation he still didn't seem to understand how serious his illness had been.

"What am I doing here?" he demanded when I came to see him. "Take me home."

"Honey, look at you." I lifted his hospital gown to show him the scar.

"I don't know why they did that. Those crazy American doctors," he answered.

Sasha was often incoherent. We believed it was merely the aftereffects from the illness. At times he was also a difficult patient. He'd pull at the tubes running into his body, and wander down the corridor by himself. When a nurse would take him by the arm to lead him back to his room, Sasha would yell at her, "Don't touch me. I want to get out of here."

At last, he was well enough to leave the hospital. We brought him home like a precious package, wrapped in a dressing gown and blankets.

We had hired a Russian woman to help with the housework and meals, and she took one look at Sasha's thin face and vowed she would quickly get the weight back on him. She went to work at the stove, permeating our home with the provoking smells of Russian specialities: piroshki, thick bowls of borsch, and *kotleti*, a fluffy-type Russian hamburger, so succulent that its juices spurt out when pricked with a fork.

Each morning she prepared a huge batch of buckwheat kasha, which we ate as a cereal and also as a side dish to lamb or duck. Sasha never failed to tell us he knew a medical professor in Moscow who cured all stomach ailments by prescribing kasha.

We pampered him, met all his needs. I went out of my way to find some new books that I thought might interest Sasha. Ever since I had known him he had been a voracious reader. Before the operation our evenings were often spent with both of us engrossed in books. To us, these evenings accentuated our common interests and how well we got on together.

Sasha rarely revealed his feelings to other people, but when we were alone he turned books into a means for an intimate discussion. "Listen to this," he'd say, reading certain paragraphs aloud to me. "I understand this so well. Do you understand it?"

The more personal a writer became, the more Sasha bared his own being. There is a phrase, "You have to eat the whole pudding before you come to the raisin." Sasha consumed each book until he found that raisin.

He used to tell me, "In Russian literature you find the native genius of the people." He quoted long passages from Pushkin, Tolstoy, and Gorki. In particular, he valued the work of Dostoevski. "No psychiatrist in the world," he would insist, "could understand the workings of the soul the way Dostoevski could."

After he returned from the hospital, I expected Sasha to

renew his pleasure in books, thinking they would relieve the boredom while I was away at work, but it was weeks before he finally picked up one of his favorites.

However, he was never able to read more than two or three pages at a time. I would find him asleep sitting up on our yellow sofa, the book still in his lap, his head back, with his mouth hanging open. I'd sit beside him, disturbed by the looseness in his face; he seemed lifeless.

On several occasions I noticed as he slept his fingers jerked. They would fly out, tapping the book, as if he were composing his own masterpiece. It was weird to see those fingers moving while the rest of his body was so inert.

His illness had struck about six months before he was expected to retire from the American Can Company. I had hoped he might get a chance to go back to work for at least a couple of months before the official retirement date, but as time went on it was obvious he didn't even have the energy to leave the house.

One day I got a call from his boss saying that he and a colleague would like to come and visit Sasha. He added they had collected some money to buy Sasha a retirement gift. Did I have any ideas what he needed?

When I got off the telephone I approached Sasha. "Your friends from the office say they miss you."

He didn't look up.

"They want to visit you, and they've collected some money to get a gift. Is there anything you really want?"

"I don't care. It doesn't matter."

He sounded disinterested. Later I tried to talk to him about the retirement, but continued to get little response. Was he hiding his feelings? After all, he had given them eighteen years of his life, and it had to be a difficult experience retiring under these circumstances.

The boss and the colleague came early one afternoon, taking

time off work for their visit. They arrived with good wishes from his other friends, and a box filled with Sasha's personal papers from his office desk.

They placed the box down on our coffee table and started emptying it . . . a calendar, telephone book, engineering books, drawings. There was also a set of fine drafting instruments stored in a velvet case, precious to Sasha because he had used these instruments since he was a young man.

Then they handed him a plastic portfolio containing retirement documents, detailing his life insurance and social security benefits.

I looked at the portfolio and thought: Is that what it's about? Eighteen years ending in one afternoon, terminated by plastic pages trimmed in black. The black trim seemed to depict the finality of it all.

They gave Sasha the gifts from the office, an electric drill and a set of screwdrivers, tools I had told the men Sasha needed. With the gifts came a card. Sasha had been popular at work and the messages on the card were kind and caring, urging Sasha to stay in touch.

"Over fifty people signed your card. We're all going to miss you, especially the women," said the boss, turning to give me a good-natured wink.

"Look what we found in your desk," continued the boss, tumbling dozens of pencils out onto our carpet. "You must have been swiping these for years. No wonder nobody else in the company could ever find any pencils."

Sasha stared at the pencils without smiling, although his boss continued to joke about them. Ever since they had arrived Sasha had been polite but cool, almost as if he didn't recognize them. I quickly brought out drinks to relieve the tension, but I knew his former colleagues were embarrassed.

The visitors searched for office gossip that might amuse Sasha, but their laughter spilled into silent gaps when Sasha looked blankly at them as they talked about certain people. Over and over again he murmured, "I don't remember him."

Of course he had to remember. He'd only been away from the office a few months. I just couldn't understand Sasha's behavior.

"Well, if we can do anything for you, just let us know," said his boss, pushing himself up from the sofa to leave.

"Thank you," said Sasha.

"Anything, anything at all," repeated the boss, glancing down at Sasha's slippers. I had a feeling he wanted to reach out and slap Sasha on the back, give him a hearty farewell, but instead he shook Sasha's hand, avoided his eyes, and left.

Before his kidney operation, Sasha appeared to have limitless energy. At sixty-five, he still looked as if he were in his early fifties. I would return from my office and moan, "I'm exhausted," but Sasha would put in an eight-hour day at the American Can Company and then look for work to do at night around the house; he was constantly refinishing furniture, painting, anything to keep busy.

I'd ask, "Aren't you tired?" and he'd say, "Tired? What's tired?" I'd laugh and tell him it was his Cossack genes that gave him the super stamina. Somehow I believed my husband would never grow old.

Sasha used to reinforce this belief by assuring me he intended to keep on working for many more years. "When I retire from the American Can Company," he contemplated, "I plan to look for another job, perhaps in engineering, or maybe I can find some remodeling work to do for other people. I can't sit around the house all day."

I therefore expected Sasha to start looking for a job as soon as he had healed from his surgery. As the months passed, though, he showed absolutely no interest in work.

He was content to stay for hours in our garden. He would search for weeds, his fingers pulling at any unwanted sign of nature, until the earth looked picture-clean. A long time ago Sasha had planted two birch trees to remind him of the birch trees in Samara that had lined the avenue leading to the estate where he was born. Now he often sat under the birch trees in our garden, detached, dreaming. I came home once to find him sitting outside in the fog, unaware his hair and clothes were drenched by the dampness in the air.

I began to get annoyed. I felt he was becoming lazy, withdrawn, was using his illness as an excuse to shirk responsibilities. By this time, I thought, he should have recovered from the operation. After all, there were thousands of people who lived an active life with one kidney.

I was also getting concerned about our financial situation. Sasha was receiving a small pension, along with his social security, but the total was less than five hundred dollars a month. I was glad I was working, and yet I knew if Sasha didn't get a job it would be a tight squeeze to meet all our expenses, especially since we wanted to send Nicky to college.

We had always tried to give Nicky the best of everything. He was attending a private high school and had shown exceptional artistic talent, winning an award three years in a row from the American Institute of Architects. Even as a young boy Nicky had been fascinated with structure and design, spending hours building model trains and complicated systems that required commendable patience.

Nicky's temperament was low-key, and when he was a small child he was inclined to be shy. To counter his shyness Sasha and I had given him accordion lessons. He became quite good with the accordion, but later complained to us that we had chosen the wrong instrument; he was, he said, far more interested in the guitar! Eventually all music was dropped for greater interests—sports and girls. He had the looks to attract the girls and the athletic ability to play a competitive game of basketball and soccer.

There was also a meditative side to Nicky. At age fourteen he wrote in a school essay: "Man is the Universe. He is the ultimate being. He contains all the knowledge in the universe. I am all of that. What is my destiny? Am I to be the enlightenment of myself and my fellow beings? Will I use my knowledge to my benefit and the benefit of others, or will I use it to destroy my fellow man?"

We saved the best of his school essays and drawings, and doted on him. We enjoyed him so much that we wanted to be a total part of his life, which, looking back, was probably wrong.

I started to needle Sasha about our wish to send Nicky to college, and how it would help if he went back to work. "You always told me that you would find another job after you left the American Can Company," I reminded him.

"All right, I'll think about getting a job."

"What do you mean you'll think about it? Look at this. This seems a good one," I insisted, pointing to a newspaper ad for a job I had circled in black ink. "You should go for an interview. Why don't you go tomorrow?"

"I'll think about it."

The next day I asked him, "Well, did you inquire about that job?"

"No."

"Why not?"

"Tomorrow. Don't rush me, Anne," he said angrily. "Maybe I'll go tomorrow."

He didn't go. So I kept underlining ads that I thought might be suitable.

Finally I demanded, "Call this man. I want to come home and find out you have done something."

Normally I wouldn't have talked to Sasha in that tone; it was contrary to our whole relationship, for we weren't the type to nag or chip away at each other. Throughout our marriage I had considered Sasha the dominant partner, the person I could depend on. He coddled me, sustained me.

All of a sudden, I saw the roles reversed. Since I was the only one working, Sasha was now dependent upon my income, my support. The more I saw him leaning on me, the more anxious I became. I wanted my husband to take control again.

I have never been what one considers a submissive person. On the contrary, my friends describe me as a woman with a strong, independent streak, and I know they're right. Yet . . . what I didn't tell my friends, and what I only admitted to myself occasionally, was that there was a vulnerable part of me that represented the child who never grew up. I wanted someone to look after me.

During an evening when my parents joined us for dinner I blurted out my fears. "I'm petrified," I acknowledged. "Financially I have to take care of the whole family, and I don't know what I am going to do."

Sasha was sitting beside me, and I knew it was unkind to speak that way in front of him but I wanted to shake him up, elicit some sort of response. My husband's face didn't change.

It was my father's reaction that astonished me. "Sasha has worked long enough," he said. "You are young. You are healthy. It's your turn."

I retreated, changing the conversation to something trivial. I was left feeling depressed, beaten down by the sense nobody—not even my parents—understood my concern.

What did my father mean? I was working. I had always worked. I wanted my father to say, "Don't worry." I had wanted him to assure me things were going to get back to the way they were. To me that meant Sasha feeling well enough to work. To me it was that logical.

I longed for our former life so badly that I ignored the fragments of strangeness surrounding Sasha's behavior.

On one job interview he went to, Sasha was asked some questions that he couldn't answer. Driving home after the interview, Sasha took off his hat and threw it out the car window.

When I asked Sasha where his hat was he replied, "I threw it out," as if that was an adequate explanation.

"What do you mean you threw it out? It was an expensive hat, and there was nothing wrong with it."

"I opened the car window, took the hat and threw it out."

"I can't believe this." I wanted to probe further, but he turned away, silencing me.

It was during this time our house was robbed. After being out for a couple of hours we returned to find the front door jimmied. Inside chests of drawers had been pulled apart, their contents strewn. The television, my jewelry, and many of our valuables were taken, including Sasha's set of drafting instruments, which he had treasured so much.

When the police arrived they suggested we prevent further burglaries by installing a wrought-iron grille over the glass panel in our front door.

The man who came to install the grille was the type of person who liked to talk as he worked. I found myself standing in the hallway with him, listening to his family problems, and then I told him about my own. I told him about Sasha's operation, his long recovery, and how I hoped my husband would soon find a job.

"Would he like to work for me?" said the man.

His offer was so unexpected it took me a minute before I responded, "Well, he might. Let me ask him."

Sasha, to my delight, was agreeable to the idea. It was only a small salary, but I felt anything would be better than Sasha stagnating at home. The job, I thought, might stir the life-juices, return Sasha to his vigorous self.

Two days after Sasha started working I received a telephone call at my office from the man who had offered to employ him. "I'm sorry to bother you," he said. "It's about your husband. Things aren't working out. When I show Sasha how to do something he acts as if he is paying attention, but when I come back half an hour later he either hasn't done anything at all, or he's made some mistake."

"He's still new at the job," I responded.

"I'm willing to take that into consideration," said the man. "Why don't you talk to him and see if there's any problem. I want to help both of you."

Toward the end of the week the man called again. "It's no use. Your husband forgets everything I tell him. I can't trust him to complete the work."

I defended Sasha. The man listened patiently. He was exceptionally kind. Anyone else would probably have fired Sasha on the first day, but he kept him for two weeks before he let him go.

It took an incident at another job to jolt me into recognizing Sasha wasn't capable of work.

A friend of mine mentioned she knew somebody who needed electrical wiring done in her house. "It's just a small job. Do you think Sasha would like to do it?"

"He might," I replied. "He's done wiring before. He once worked for Bethlehem Steel, installing wiring on a ship."

This time I questioned Sasha carefully. "Do you feel you can handle the job? Are you well enough to do it?"

"Sure I can handle it," he said, his familiar confident self. "It will be no problem."

He left in the morning to go to the woman's house, and didn't return until late afternoon. When he walked in our front door I could see by the tightness in his face things hadn't gone well. He looked befuddled.

"Did you finish the job?" I asked.

"No. I'll have to go back tomorrow." He folded his body into a chair, leaned his head back and closed his eyes.

"Did it go all right though? Could you manage it?" My nervousness played with my stomach.

"It was okay," he said.

It wasn't okay. That night the woman rang and complained

Sasha hadn't done what she wanted. Again, I made excuses, gave assurances.

The following morning Sasha wanted to return to the woman's house. I didn't know what to do. The only thing I could think of was to send Nicky with him, in case he could assist his father.

They were gone for many hours. When they came back Nicky waited until Sasha wasn't in the room and then he said quietly, "Oh Mom, you should have seen what Papa did. It was a real mess. I had to take the wiring apart and redo it."

I listened to Nicky's words, and it was then I acknowledged the root of my uneasiness. If my son could do a job he had never done before, why couldn't Sasha handle it? Why was it taking him so long to recover?

I had questioned the doctor before about Sasha, only to hear the stereotyped reply, "He's recuperating. At his age he went through a serious operation. Just give him time."

Time. Months have a way of speeding past. Three months. Five months. The doctor gave Sasha vitamin-B shots but they didn't help. Seven months. We changed doctors, but all I could tell each doctor was that my husband was lethargic, forgetful, moody—all natural symptoms, I was told, considering what he had been through.

It seems the medical profession responds best in an emergency, but when symptoms drag on sluggishly, when there's a flat line without any urgent decline, then the doctors don't always know how to react.

I knew what they were thinking: They saw a young wife trying to shake up an old tree trunk and make him function again like a sapling. They were cemented to demographics and their medical books, while I was attached to real life; we were functioning from two different places. To them Sasha appeared to be a man getting on in years and they didn't look any further, while I considered Sasha extraordinarily young for his age, who only a few months ago had spark and vitality. I couldn't accept the idea such vitality could be dislodged so dramatically.

Sasha, himself, never seemed concerned about his slow recovery, and nor did it worry him when I used to tell him, "Sasha, you're forgetting things." If I chided him for neglecting to tell me somebody called, or not paying a bill, he would just smile and agree his memory wasn't very good any more, and dismiss the subject as unimportant.

I knew something wasn't quite right. Yet, it never occurred to me anything was seriously wrong. I had been assured the kidney operation had been successful and Sasha was in good physical shape. I simply felt the doctors were ignoring some small factor that would return Sasha to full health. Maybe he needed more vitamins, another pill, a special diet.

We chose, instead, another doctor. Sasha took a liking to this doctor because he wore a bow tie. For Sasha, the bow tie was like a key to a club; to him it meant the doctor was a gentleman, and could be trusted.

After this doctor had seen Sasha a couple of times he suggested we visit a neurologist.

"Why do we need to go to a neurologist?" I asked.

"I think it would be wise to get some additional tests done," he replied, handing me a piece of paper with a name scribbled on it. "I recommend this man."

The neurologist asked me to sit in the waiting room while he examined Sasha. They were gone for over half an hour and when they came out Sasha looked tired and angry.

"Let's go home," Sasha said sharply.

"I need to talk to you, Mrs. Bashkiroff," intervened the doctor. "Could you persuade your husband to wait outside for a minute?"

I picked up my handbag and coat. "I won't be long, darling," I said casually to Sasha.

The neurologist closed his office door and walked over to his side of the desk. "I've given your husband a series of number and word-association tests," he said, his manner blunt. "It's just as I suspected. Your husband has presenile dementia."

The words were transmitted coldly, abruptly. There was no preparation, no easing into the diagnosis. I felt as though the doctor had taken a bucket of ice-cold water and thrown it over my head.

"*Presenile dementia.*" It was the first time I had heard those two words together. To me, "senile" meant the loss of mental facilities due to old age, and "dementia" meant crazy. Was this doctor telling me my husband had become senile and would end up in a lunatic asylum? Fear whipped my mind, and it seemed forever before I could ask, "What can be done?"

"To be honest with you, nothing. There is no cure, and I'm afraid it will get progressively worse. You're going to have to accept the fact your husband will deteriorate."

I stared at the doctor's professional mask. His emotionless face gave me no comfort, and I wanted to scream: Be human. Help me. You've given me a death warrant. You've ended two lives with two words. How can you be so brusque, so unfeeling?

Perhaps after a time doctors lose compassion, or forget how to show compassion, or maybe some of them need to remain aloof to preserve their own mental health. Whatever the reasons or excuses, their emotional distance at such a time only intensifies the shock.

Shock . . . shattering all of me as the doctor noted—oh so clinically—"Before long he won't be able to take care of himself, and you will probably have to place him somewhere."

Place him? What was this doctor talking about? Sasha had only a slight loss of memory; he might forget to keep appointments, or give me telephone messages, but they were little irritations, minor nuisances in our lives. I could live with them. Place him in a home? My God!

As I sat there, aghast, listening to the neurologist, Sasha

pushed open the door. "What's going on here?" he demanded.
"Let's get out of this place."

"Sasha, please," I said. "I'll only be a few more minutes."
I got up, took his hand, and led him out the door.

"By the way," said the doctor as I came back into his office.
"How did you get here?"

"By car," I replied, thinking it was an odd question.

"Did your husband drive?"

"Yes, he always does. I don't drive."

The doctor's expression changed. A firmness set into his
mouth as he said, almost harshly, "You must realize Sasha
shouldn't drive any more. He's dangerous to himself and to
others."

"How am I to get home?" Everything was collapsing about
me.

"He mustn't drive," repeated the doctor. "Nor should you
leave him at home alone."

So easy for the neurologist: Orders handed out like a
prescription for cough medicine. Swallow in one gulp. Change
your ways, end your lives. Don't drive any more. My God!

Sasha charged into the room again. "Let's go," he ordered,
and in Russian he added, "*Sookin sin!*" (son-of-a-bitch).

We left. I held on tightly to Sasha and didn't say a word to
him. I thought to myself, "Screw you, doctor. You're wrong. My
husband is not senile or crazy."

Sasha drove us home.

Chapter 4

IN SICKNESS AND IN HEALTH

For a long while I didn't believe the doctor's diagnosis. I had left his office in a rush, upset and bewildered. The doctor never called me back to say, "Let's sit down and talk about the diagnosis and what it will mean to your family."

He dropped me. And I dropped him. I went to another doctor to seek another opinion. I searched my head for excuses about Sasha's head. On our journey from Buenos Aires to San Francisco, Sasha had hit his forehead against some metal in the ship's engine room, cutting his skull so it bled. Maybe that incident had caused a problem.

Maybe it was a nonmalignant tumor. Surely it was something that could be corrected? Tell me anything, but don't tell me there is no cure.

Each time I heard a doctor say to me, "Mrs. Bashkiroff, nothing is going to help. Eventually you're going to have to place your husband in a nursing home," I decided to make an appointment with somebody else.

I realized Sasha was sick, but I couldn't perceive the future being worse than the present. I couldn't imagine Sasha deteriorating to the point where I had to put him in a home. I could only envision taking care of him and living out our lives together—not happily ever after—but at least together.

I started reading trashy magazines because they sometimes printed news about phenomenal cures. I would cut these articles out, thinking, I'll try that. I was prepared to do anything, go anywhere. If the magazine mentioned a medication, I'd call the doctor and ask, "Do you think we could give this to Sasha?" The answer was usually an empthatic no.

Even though I was working for a hospital, knew a little bit about medicine, and supposedly am an intelligent woman, I refused to accept that Sasha's illness was degenerative and irreversible.

I went through at least seven doctors—two neurologists and five internists. It was a struggle to persuade Sasha to see these physicians. I'd call from my office and say, "Darling, I'm leaving work early. Can you pick me up in an hour?"

"I'd be glad to. Why are you leaving work?"

"We're going to the doctor's."

"Aren't you feeling well?" There would be genuine concern in his voice.

"It isn't for me. It's for you."

Sasha's tone would change immediately. "There's nothing wrong with me. I'm not going."

I'd cajole him. "Go just to please me. You know how I worry about you. I won't have to worry if you go."

"All right, all right," he'd finally say, submitting to my appeals. "For your sake I'll see a doctor."

The next problem was keeping him at the doctor's office. He could never understand why doctors didn't honor the appointed time. After waiting two minutes he'd say, "Where is that doctor? To hell with it, I'm leaving."

I would have to rush after him, try to persuade him to be more patient.

I sometimes tricked Sasha into seeing a doctor by pretending the appointment was for me. I had to resort to these tricks because it was never explained to Sasha he had presenile dementia. I never told him. Neither did the doctors.

Looking back, I believe this was one of the greatest mistakes we made. If we had been honest with Sasha, especially in the early stages of his illness, I am sure it would have lessened his confusion about what was happening to him. However, I wasn't in any state to be honest with Sasha, because I wasn't even being honest with myself. I hadn't come to terms with the diagnosis. My primary response was denial.

Initially, I didn't ask the doctors enough questions. I felt if I didn't talk about it, then the whole problem would go away. On the other hand, the doctors didn't help the situation because they didn't volunteer information that might have forced me to be more realistic about how to handle Sasha's illness. They loaded me with the diagnosis, and stressed there was no cure, but they didn't give me any suggestions on how to take care of Sasha during the early stages of the illness, and they didn't adequately explain the difficult emotional and practical problems I would have to face as the disease progressed.

And although some doctors were kind to me personally, I felt that too many of them treated my husband crudely. They never attempted to talk to him about his symptoms; in many ways they seemed to treat him as if he were a machine that had broken down, a machine to be placed in storage because he was no longer of any use to society. What's more, although I behaved stupidly and irrationally by refusing to accept that Sasha's illness was incurable, this form of denial by family members who are presented with a dire diagnosis is not unusual, and I think doctors should encourage follow-up treatment for families under these circumstances. If a doctor had offered to talk to us, as a family unit, on a continuing basis it would have helped enormously. Instead, they all just gave me a "sentence of despair" and then, because there was no cure, didn't attempt to see us again.

When I first heard the term "presenile dementia" it didn't

make much sense to me. Today, I am aware of these facts: The word "dementia" refers to progressive intellectual decline and memory loss. Presenile dementia and senile dementia are the same condition, although doctors sometimes use the term "presenile" when the patient is under sixty-five.

There are several forms of dementia, but Alzheimer's disease appears to account for about fifty percent of the irreversible dementias. Alzheimer's disease is not a normal part of aging, and although the disease is far more prevalent after sixty, Alzheimer's has also been seen in people as young as twenty-eight. Dementia can happen to anyone; there are no social or racial lines, and brilliant people can become impaired just as severely as anybody else.

Sasha was given a CAT scan, which showed moderate cerebral atrophy, or so-called shrinkage of the brain. This can be indicative of Alzheimer's disease, but many researchers feel the correlation between atrophy and Alzheimer's is not strong enough to make a definitive diagnosis.

The diagnosis for Alzheimer's can only be made by observing the symptoms and by eliminating all other possible causes of senile dementia. Unfortunately, in Sasha's case, this process of elimination created confusion. During the first few years of Sasha's illness not one doctor mentioned to me that Sasha's senile dementia might be Alzheimer's disease. I was given several other possible explanations for his dementia, and it wasn't until Sasha had reached the last stages of his disease that I finally was informed he probably had Alzheimer's because he then showed the characteristic symptoms.

Alzheimer's is the fourth leading cause of death in the United States. The disease is named after Alois Alzheimer, a German neurologist who first described it in 1906. Practically no research was conducted on Alzheimer's until the 1960s, and it's only recently that there have been major advances in research. However, Alzheimer's is still a little-understood disorder. At the moment there is no cure, and the doctors can't stop its progression.

We do know Alzheimer's occurs in the nerve cells of the cerebral cortex, and in particular the hippocampus. Nerve fibers and filaments are left in tangles, and groups of nerve endings degenerate into what are called plaques. These plaques and tangles ultimately kill the nerve cells; the more lesions in a person's brain, the greater the disturbance in intellectual functioning.

It is difficult to predict how each person will behave. Some patients become volatile and violent, while others become extremely inert. The onset of Alzheimer's is usually gradual, with the first signs being short-term memory loss and impaired concentration. In the early stages the personality changes can also be mild, so it's easy to delude oneself into thinking the symptoms won't become severe; the patient won't get as bad as someone else with a similar disorder.

For seven years after I was given the original diagnosis of presenile dementia I kept Sasha at home. For seven years I observed the step-by-step rotting of my husband's brain cells. During all that time I thought I could cope, but as Sasha's brain deteriorated, so did our lives.

One day we met a friend from Buenos Aires, whom we hadn't seen for a long time. He had known Sasha as a boisterous, outspoken person, and I could tell he was surprised to see Sasha now so listless. I should have taken him aside and told him, "Sasha's not well." I didn't say anything. I didn't want to answer difficult questions. Many people mistakingly think dementia is a mental illness. I found it hard to tell people Sasha was a man who was literally losing his mind, not out of his mind.

The man ordered us cocktails before dinner. Sasha was on medication and wasn't supposed to take any alcohol, but I thought one drink wouldn't do any harm.

The man ordered a second round. "Honey, no more," I said to Sasha.

"What's this, Sasha?" noted the man, giving me a disdainful look. "Since when do you allow your wife to boss you around?"

It was a foolish remark that shouldn't have hurt me as much as it did, and yet it was the kind of comment I kept hearing and sensing. I found it more and more difficult to socialize, or go out to any public place.

I had always been so proud of Sasha's intelligence, but now I found myself covering up for my husband so people wouldn't ridicule him. If somebody spoke to Sasha he'd often reply with a totally inappropriate comment, or look at me with startled eyes and not say anything at all. I'd intervene in conversations, jump in and give opinions for him. Every time I shielded him, I could see people look at each other as if to say, "What's the matter with her?"

Even our friends who knew what was the matter, who should have accepted Sasha's illness, began to pull away from us. It became obvious Sasha's dementia made them feel awkward. People stopped asking us out, and began to make excuses why they couldn't come to our house. I discovered a distressing reality: It's much easier for friends to come to your aid if you have a short-term problem. There are few people capable of dealing with a long-term tragedy. It's too emotionally demanding.

We stayed home. We lived in an ever-diminishing world.

During the week, Sasha drove me to work. I ignored the advice of the neurologist who said Sasha shouldn't handle a car any more because I felt such drastic action wasn't necessary. As far as I could detect, Sasha was driving the same as he always did, not any better, and not any worse.

In truth, during all the years I knew Sasha, he had never been a good driver. All his frustrations came out when he was behind the wheel. He tooted the horn like a maniac, believed in his own road rules, and collected tickets as if they were souvenirs of his travels.

I had never learned to drive because I had thought Sasha would always be around to take me anywhere I wished. I had believed there was no need for me to learn.

A few months after Sasha was diagnosed as having senile dementia he had to renew his driver's license. I arranged for a tutor to help Sasha on the written test. I didn't tell the tutor about Sasha's illness and the tutor never asked why Sasha had so much difficulty remembering the rules.

To renew his license Sasha had to fill out an application form that included the question, "Within the last three years, have you experienced a lapse of consciousness, or had any disease, disorder or disability which affects your ability to exercise reasonable and ordinary control in operating a motor vehicle?"

Sasha wrote no. Not only did he not realize he had a disorder that might affect his ability to drive, but he probably didn't understand the question.

Sasha managed to pass the test. Because he had developed cataracts he was only given a limited license. When it came time to renew the license again, I got another tutor. This time he passed the written test, but failed the actual driving test. What's more, during the eye exam it was discovered the cataracts were worse.

"Did you know," the examiner said to Sasha, "you are blind in one eye?"

If I had been wise, I would have hidden Sasha's car keys right then. I should have understood it was dangerous for him to be on the road, but Sasha wasn't the only one who was partly blind.

I felt the car was Sasha's only lifeline; driving was the one thing he could still do that gave him independence. I thought Sasha couldn't function without a car, which is ridiculous because one can function without many things.

Today, I realize so many of my actions and reactions were

mishandled. My values were faulty, and the things that I believed to be important weren't important at all. I kept batting my head against the wall, wanting the wall to give.

In my desperation to renew his driver's license, I took Sasha to see our opthalmologist. I didn't mention the dementia, so the eye doctor concluded Sasha's right eye was strong enough to compensate for the bad eye, and he should be allowed to drive. Armed with the recommendation from the opthalmologist, and with the help of additional tutoring, Sasha renewed his license once again.

Sasha had always been a helpful man, and for a long time I was able to keep him busy at home while I went to work. He did a little shopping, some cleaning, and took over the washing and ironing. Each job took him hours to complete, filling up most of the day.

I only gave him minor chores, things that didn't matter if he couldn't manage them. If he broke a dish it was nothing; if he forgot to mail the insurance check it might be critical.

Although Sasha could still recall his childhood in Russia vividly, his short-term memory often failed him. For this reason I developed a habit of repeating myself. Before I left for work, I'd say, "Darling, can you put the casserole in the oven at three o'clock?"

"Fine," he'd answer, acting as if the request had been absorbed.

I'd call midmorning to see if he was all right. Casually I'd ask, "Sasha, did you remember you had to start the oven at three o'clock?"

"You never told me."

"All right. Please, will you put the casserole in at three o'clock?"

I got accustomed to repeating myself not just two or three times, but at least ten times. This habit became so automatic I would say things over and over again to my son as well as Sasha. I drove Nicky wild. Yet by this time the need for repetition was a fearful response to an unpredictable environment.

Sasha began to misplace objects, misjudge things. I couldn't assume he had unplugged the iron, or turned off the stove.

My neighbor and friend, Doris Dunbar, was standing with me in my kitchen when Sasha was preparing coffee in our drip-pot. We watched in silence as Sasha poured orange juice instead of water into the pot.

Doris was also with me on the day Sasha decided to hang up the saucepans to dry on the clothesline outside. Sasha didn't seem perturbed that the clothespins wouldn't snap onto the handles of the saucepans; for several minutes he fumbled with the clothespins, a blank look on his face as the saucepans kept falling to the ground.

Another time, when it was raining heavily, he took the garden hose and watered down the already soaked sidewalk.

Although Doris witnessed several of these incidents with me, I never discussed them with her. I had told her he had an illness, but I was still not willing to admit to her or to myself that Sasha's mind was steadily unraveling. Dementia has a certain stigma in society, and I was ashamed of the illness, ashamed of Sasha . . . ashamed of my own behavior.

All his life Sasha had been fastidiously neat. Now, after he shaved, there were pockets of stubble that his razor had missed. Knowing how important Sasha's appearance had been to him I tried to assist him, refusing to allow the illness to lower the high standards Sasha once followed.

"Can I shave you?" I'd offer.

"No, don't touch me. If you don't like my face, don't look at it," Sasha would reply defensively. "Go look at the doctors at your hospital. I'm sure they're handsome."

I think by this time Sasha knew his mind was slipping, which made him cling even more to his strength of will.

Occasionally, after a great deal of protest, I did shave him. I also cut his hair, because he refused to go to the barber. I bought electric hair clippers. It took me a while to get used to them. Once, I moved the clippers too quickly, and slashed off too much hair on one side of Sasha's head.

Sasha, who had been holding a hand mirror, stood up in a rage, yelling, "Leave me alone. Leave me alone."

"Honey, please sit down. I'll do it again. I'll make it look better."

"No, leave me alone. Don't come near me."

For the rest of the week Sasha walked around with the hair on one side of his head too short, the other side too long.

I now realize it was stupid to have worried so much about Sasha's appearance. So what if I gave him a rotten haircut? So what if he had stubble on his chin? He could have grown a beard. At that time I didn't understand these problems were petty, and that soon I would face situations far more critical.

I got caught by the joke that goes: Things can't get worse. Then they do.

Bad events piled on top of one another, making my load heavier and heavier until I wondered how much I could handle; yesterday's load now seemed light, tomorrow's burden seemed impossible.

My father developed cancer of the lung. At first we thought radiation treatment had controlled the cancer, but within six months the cancer spread, and he had to be hospitalized.

Two days after he entered the hospital, my mother went into a catatonic state. The doctors couldn't find a physical cause for my mother's problem, but I theorized my father's illness terrified her so much she escaped into a coma, just as years earlier she'd faint to avoid unpleasant circumstances.

Fortunately, her coma was brief. My parents had been placed in opposite rooms on the same floor of the hospital. I'd get out of the elevator holding Sasha's hand, and hear my mother calling, "Anne, Anne." Then my father would see me and beckon. I didn't know which room to go into first.

Several years earlier my mother had suffered a stroke that left her right side partly paralyzed. This time the doctors informed me she had high blood pressure, a weak heart, and was a candidate for another serious stroke. My mother and father, they said, were not well enough to look after themselves. They suggested I place my parents in a home.

I had always respected my parents' privacy and hated the idea, and now the task, of sifting through their personal papers and belongings. Haphazardly, I dismantled their apartment, gave things to neighbors, to anyone who would take them. Material goods were losing their importance.

I arranged for my parents to go to the same convalescent home, but my mother insisted my father be placed on a different floor. Basically their marriage was never a good one, and she chose this period in their lives to permanently reject him. Every time he came looking for her in the convalescent home she refused to talk to him, and wouldn't even let him stay near her.

I later settled my mother in the Jewish Home for the Aged. I had planned for my father to follow her there as soon as there was another opening, but he died in February 1972, a month after my mother moved away from him.

In the continuing storm Nicky was my rainbow. He won a scholarship to Rensselaer Polytechnic Institute in Troy, New York, where he planned to study architecture. I didn't like the idea of him leaving home, and yet I was determined Sasha's illness wasn't going to spoil my son's future.

When Sasha was first diagnosed as having presenile dementia Nicky was only fifteen years old. Initially, because I didn't accept Sasha's diagnosis, I wasn't able to discuss the consequences of the illness with my son. And as time went on, I still didn't have the foresight to sit down and talk to Nicky about what we should do as a family when Sasha's disease became worse. We simply dealt with each day as it came.

Sasha had always been a strict disciplinarian, and I don't think it was easy for Nicky to be a "regular American boy" in a home where his father was not only older than most parents, but also maintained his foreignness and old-world manners and concepts. Sasha's illness only made things worse for Nicky. We tiptoed around Sasha, allowing him to dictate to us because we weren't wise enough to take control. I'd tell Nicky, "Don't do this, it upsets your Dad." If Nicky was late for dinner, Sasha would refuse to eat. "Nicky, come at this time," I'd say. "Go at this time." Nicky yo-yoed to our commands. For his sake, it was just as well he left for college.

I wanted to give Nicky a treasured memory for his graduation party. My son was a romanticist. He had been suckled on fanciful tales about his father's life in Russia, and had grown up appreciating the fine things in life, not just in art and literature, but also in good food and good manners. We had tried to teach him to live without sham, but with social grace.

I recommended Nicky take his girlfriend and five other couples to Alexis, the most exclusive restaurant in San Francisco at that time. I had known Mr. Alexis for years, and he assured me he would give the teenagers a wonderful evening.

Sasha's handmade tuxedo from the Orient had been altered to fit Nicky, and with the tuxedo Nicky wore a new silk, ruffled shirt. My son had inherited the fine-honed looks of his father, as well as his aristocratic bearing. He was the same height as Sasha and had his coloring, hazel eyes and light brown hair. There was a certain sensuality in Nicky's face and there was no doubt young women found him alluring. As he left for his graduation dinner I thought Nicky looked undeniably handsome.

A parent's sleep can be easily broken. I woke up and looked at the clock: 2:30 A.M. Nicky hadn't come home yet, and for a few minutes I lay in bed thinking what every mother thinks. Supposing there had been an accident? I got up and telephoned the parents of Nicky's girlfriend.

"Don't worry," said the mother. "Nicky was here but he left

about fifteen minutes ago, and should be at your home any second. He's not feeling well."

"What do you mean he's not feeling well?"

"Oh, I guess he had a little too much to drink."

"What?" I was amazed at the casualness of this mother.

Just then I heard a commotion at the front door. I went downstairs to find Nicky hanging limply on the arms of his two male friends. His tuxedo and ruffled shirt were wet with vomit.

His two friends dragged him upstairs to his room, explaining Nicky had ordered several bottles of champagne in the restaurant. By this time Sasha was also awake, and he found out from the boys that they had left our car about a mile away since Nicky was in no state to drive. Sasha decided to leave at once and retrieve the car.

I didn't know whether to worry more about Sasha going out in the middle of the night, or my son making awful strangling noises behind the bathroom door.

I focused my attention—and anger—on Nicky. When his friends left, so did my control. "How could you do this?" I shouted at Nicky. He stood before me naked to the waist, his ruined shirt at his feet.

"How could you?" I repeated, and suddenly I swung at him. I hit him as hard as I could in the face. Then I hit him again. All the anger I couldn't express about Sasha's illness I now released on Nicky's drunkenness. It was something if I could have undone, I would have undone.

Nicky began to cry. I put him to bed, weeping inwardly myself, ashamed of my actions and yet full of self-pity. I had planned such a beautiful evening. Why did he spoil it?

When Sasha came back I was still justifying my feelings. "How could he do this to us? I hit him."

"What did you do?"

"I hit him."

"Don't you ever do that again." Sasha was furious with me. "This happens to young boys," he went on. "The first time I got drunk I was Nick's age. Boys have to experiment. Don't you ever hit him again."

I was stunned. I couldn't believe Sasha was telling me off. Even more important I couldn't believe he had enough power of reasoning to argue with me. He spoke with such cold understanding. He sounded so *normal!*

This was the man I knew. If Sasha could argue with me, then he couldn't be that sick. I became excited. The doctors had to be wrong. That evening, and too many other evenings, I told myself if I found another doctor he'd say Sasha was okay.

This is the insidious thing about the illness. In the early stages of the disease a person can act fine one day and terrible the next. If friends saw Sasha during the time he acted normally they would tell me, "I don't know what you're talking about. Sasha seems all right to me."

I sometimes wondered if I was imagining problems . . . or if I was the one who was strange. And then the day would come again when I would attempt a conversation and it would end in nonsense.

So I lived on a see-saw, never knowing what to expect.

The years went by, punctuated by one small crisis after another. I lived each day as if it were darkened by heavy clouds; I kept wishing it would rain and there would be relief, but the days only seemed to get gloomier.

I spent a lot of time living vicariously through Nicky. I wrote to him as often as I could, agonized about any problem he had with college, rejoiced in any success.

Sasha also wrote to Nicky. Interestingly his letters appeared lucid:

"Dear Pusska," one began,

Somehow it is kind of lonely not to see you or hear your voice, but of course there is nothing that can be done. The only thing is to hope that you will write often and December will soon be here.

I don't say much, but I have all the time thoughts, mostly about you. I am proud that you have ambition, which I never had. I am convinced now that you have talent and ability, which will take you far, and you will be another Bashkiroff that has succeeded, like the first Nicholas.

I love you,
Your father.

Take care of yourself.

At first Nicky returned our letters eagerly, but as he became more involved with college and his own life, there would be long periods when we didn't hear from him.

I would get upset. Sasha would get irrational. "Disown him," he'd say, on finding the mail box empty. "He's no longer my son."

I knew it was the illness talking.

Each small crisis came without warning. Although I knew it wasn't completely safe for Sasha to drive a car, I had lulled myself into thinking he was all right if he drove around familiar streets.

It was my own form of Russian roulette. Each morning when Sasha took me to work, I'd stand on the corner and wait until he had completed the U-turn, because I was afraid he might forget how to make a U-turn. I'd go to my office and give him five minutes. Then I'd call home to make sure he had arrived back safely.

If he didn't answer my body would fill with fear. I'd keep calling, hoping he was out in the garden and just hadn't heard the telephone. My nerves wouldn't rest until I knew he was all right.

One day Sasha called me. His voice was disjointed. He said he had taken the car to get groceries, made a U-turn, and somebody had bumped into him.

I raced out of the office.

By the time I reached the scene of the accident, a policeman was already talking to the woman driver of the sportscar Sasha had slammed into. The policeman and woman were laughing and I saw them exchange telephone numbers. Great, I thought, they're flirting while I'm at my wit's end.

We were lucky. The cars weren't badly damaged, and nobody was hurt. What's more, the young policeman, having apparently succeeded in getting a date, was so pleased with himself he told us, "I'm not going to give your husband a ticket because it will go against his driving record, but you must promise me you'll call up your insurance company."

I thought, oh brother, if you only knew the true story.

The accident made me finally wake up to the risk I was taking in letting Sasha drive. God forbid, he could have killed somebody!

The next day I spoke to some friends and asked them to come into our garage and take the car away. I explained I would keep Sasha busy so he wouldn't know what was happening. They resisted. They couldn't imagine taking the car without Sasha's permission. The situation was embarrassing for them because they had trouble comprehending what the illness was doing to us. I begged them. I didn't want any money, I said. I just wanted to get rid of the car.

Sasha didn't miss the car until several hours after it was gone.

"Where's the car?" he said, coming back from the garage.

"Honey, don't you remember? We took it to a garage to have it fixed."

"I don't remember giving it to anybody to be fixed."

Why did he chose this day to remember things correctly? This was one occasion when I wanted him to have no memory. Yet the disease always had the last word. When you wanted him to be abnormal he was all too normal.

So the search for the car began. He'd walk around the block

several times a day. He'd get up in the middle of the night and stare at the empty garage.

"I don't understand it. I don't understand it," he kept saying.

Finally, I offered another lie. "You sold the car to Joe Thompson." I invented some man's name, because I was concerned if he knew who really took the car he'd go to their house and demand it back.

"What are you talking about?" replied Sasha, more distressed than ever. "I never sold the car."

"Darling, we were sitting here together and you said it was an old car and you didn't want it."

It was terrible to lie, terrible to watch my husband's confusion. Eventually he forgot about the car, but it took a long time.

From then on Sasha walked everywhere, and it became his habit to visit a small neighborhood grocery store every day. One afternoon I happened to go into the store with Sasha. The owner, Ned, pulled me aside and whispered, "Do you know your husband owes me for cigars?"

"How could he?" I said. "He always has enough money on him to pay for them."

Ned looked pained. "He puts the cigars in his pocket." I felt shame, as if it were I who had been caught stealing.

"Please," I implored him. "Don't bother my husband. Count how many cigars he takes. I will come every day and pay you."

I never forgot the grocery man's kindness. He must have known something was wrong with Sasha and was considerate enough not to call the police. He allowed me to keep my pride.

Not everyone was so tactful. There was an incident with a handyman I hired to build a cupboard in Nicky's room. He, too, noticed Sasha was sick. He waited until he saw Sasha sleeping on the sofa, and then called me into Nicky's bedroom. He didn't touch me, but he came so close I felt uncomfortable.

"You're too young a woman to have to put up with this," he said.

"Put up with what?" He had me backed into a wall. He was

short and solid, a walrus of a man. His face had drops of sweat on it.

"Your husband—what's the matter with him?"

"That's none of your business," I replied sharply.

"If you ever get lonely, let me know."

I could feel his breath. I didn't want Sasha to wake up and hear us, so I kept my voice low, but my remarks were cutting. The man moved aside.

For many months Sasha and I hadn't been sexually intimate. It wasn't that Sasha wasn't capable; his physical desire for sex was as strong as ever, but every time Sasha approached me I said no.

When I turned away from him in bed Sasha would complain, "You hate me."

"I love you. I truly love you," I would assure him.

Yet this was one thing I couldn't do for him. I would kiss him. I would hug him. I could sit for hours stroking his hair, his face, comforting him in a complete nurturing way until he often fell asleep in my arms . . . but I couldn't bring myself to the act of sex.

Along with altering Sasha, the disease had also permanently altered our relationship. My husband was not the Sasha I had married and in many ways he didn't even act like a man; he had become childlike. I had been turned into a parent rather than a wife. I was left with only the desire to take care of him, not to make love to him.

During this whole time I rarely cried. Then one day Sasha called me at my office and said something was stuck.

"Sasha, what are you trying to do?" I asked, because he wasn't making sense.

"I'm washing clothes, and I'm having trouble."

"Why?"

"I don't know. It got stuck."

It was a busy day at the office, and I didn't have much time to deal with Sasha on the telephone. "Just leave it alone," I said. "I'll look after it when I get home."

An hour later I called him back.

"I can't talk to you now," Sasha said. He sounded desperate. "There's water everywhere."

I called a cab.

I found Sasha in the kitchen lying under the sink, clutching a wrench. The pipes were undone and water covered the whole kitchen floor. Sasha looked pale and scared.

"What do you think you're doing?" I screamed at him.

"Can't you see what I'm doing? I'm fixing it."

My kitchen was a disaster. I knew I would have to call a plumber and that meant I would have to stay home from the office one more day. Every little incident seemed like a monumental calamity. Sasha was a wreck. I was a wreck. Suddenly I became hysterical.

I banged my hand on the table. "Dear God, what am I going to do? Dear God! Help me somebody, help me!"

I said crazy things. And then I cried like crazy.

That evening I played one of our favorite Russian gypsy records. The music was powerful, joyous, and for a moment I felt better. I thought, "It's not the end of life for me. Something good has got to happen."

Chapter 5

THE DECISION

For six years the changes in Sasha's personality were slow enough for me to absorb, but in the seventh year the deterioration became so rapid I felt as if somebody had given us a mighty shove off a sheer cliff.

"What time is it?" I asked Sasha one day.

He carefully studied the face of his watch. "Thirteen," he answered.

"What do you mean thirteen?"

"It's after twelve, so it has to be thirteen."

"Do you realize what you're saying?" I said, alarmed.

"Count for yourself," insisted Sasha. "Look: ten, eleven, twelve, thirteen. There you are."

On another day, I asked him to sign some checks. Sasha picked up a pen, started to write, and then stopped, his face sheepish. "Is this right?"

He had only managed three letters, the writing stranger than a child's first attempt with a pen.

"I don't believe this. Don't you even know how to sign your name?"

I took hold of his hand and tried to guide it, my grip and my attitude rough. "You can *write*, can't you? This is awful!" My tone was derisive. "What on earth is happening to you?"

Sasha seemed oblivious to his own decay but to me the illness was suddenly becoming too evident, too destructive, defacing Sasha indiscriminately. Before my eyes, I could see parts of him being amputated, not limbs but something even worse . . . his ability to reason, to tell the time, to write his name, for heaven's sake! I thought: Oh Lord, what part of the brain will go next?

I pulled the check out of Sasha's hand and ripped it up. As time went on I found myself becoming more impatient with him. There was a constant pressure of stress and anxiety against my inner walls and unfortunately I sometimes released this pressure by taking it out on Sasha.

Every now and then I thought I detected a hurt look on Sasha's face when he heard the sharpness of my anger. My conscience would cringe because although I hated the illness, and hated my predicament, I also never stopped loving my husband. If anything, I loved him more deeply because he had become so helpless.

If I had known it was natural to be angry it would have helped. I needed somebody to explain it was all part of my own survival process, to explain that just as Sasha rocked between being confused one minute, and perfectly okay the next, I was also suffering from my own bewildered reactions to the disease.

I didn't have anybody to guide me. At that time there were no support groups for families of brain-damaged victims. At that time the families had not started to speak out about their problems, so there wasn't any publicity in the papers or magazines about Alzheimer's disease. For the most part, the general public didn't even know anything about this disease. I was on my own.

The physicians had warned me, "You'll have to place him in a home," but they hadn't told me exactly what it would be like to witness a human brain slowly disintegrate. Nobody had prepared me for the piecemeal torture.

I was still under the impression Sasha could somehow control his illness. I believed he wasn't trying hard enough. I blamed him when things went wrong, instead of blaming the illness. I lived in fear and in ignorance.

Every day, all day, it was a senseless cycle: Sasha would leave our San Francisco home and walk the four blocks to the bus stop. Pacing the sidewalk his expression remained vacant until the bus passengers were dropped off, and then he would stare solemnly at each person, hoping for recognition.

He'd wait for over half an hour, intent only on following the rhythm of the buses as they rumbled along the route, believing I had to be on one of them. Then he would return home, but because he had no concept of time he would soon be back, a fixture on a street corner, obsessed by a bus stop that had become his safety strap to me.

The waiting, and the walking back and forth from the house, six to ten times a day, exhausted him. At the end of the day after I had finished work I knew what to expect when I got off the bus. There was a clinging sadness in his eyes from the hours of searching, and the tiredness was so obvious his skin would be colorless.

Sasha's first words were always, "Where have you been? Where were you?"

Over and over again I tried to explain I had been at work, that he shouldn't expect me until late afternoon. Such reasoning was beyond him.

On several occasions, when Sasha grew particularly weary waiting for me, he walked the two miles to the hospital where I worked. Strangely, he never got lost.

I remember being in the middle of a board meeting and hearing a commotion at the door. "Sasha's here," someone said. I got up as Sasha came toward me, his mind and clothes in disarray.

"You can't stay here," I said, embarrassed in front of my colleagues. I held his hand as I called for a cab to take us home, and he clung to my fingers, cheerful because I was now with him. I had to leave him at home, return to the office, return to wondering what he would do next.

When he wasn't waiting at the bus stop, or arriving at my office, he was on the telephone. Not just once, but dozens of times a day.

"Did you decide to spend the night?" Sasha would say, when he called.

"What are you talking about? It's ten o'clock in the morning, I just left you."

"That's what you say."

"Please dear, I'll be home soon."

I would hang up, but ten minutes later Sasha would be on the line again. "Why aren't you home?" he'd repeat. The unrelenting routine lasted well over a year. Because my co-workers knew what was wrong, my job was never challenged. Only my sanity.

At home he would search for his mother, who had been dead for years.

"Where is she?" he'd cry out, going from room to room.

"I can't understand why she didn't call if she wasn't going to come?" Sasha would say.

"Honey, you've had a bad dream." I would lead him to the sofa and sit him down. "Your mother's dead."

As he became more irrational, I became more unnerved. It was like observing the breaking up of an elaborate puzzle; every now and then there would be another part of his personality missing.

At around six o'clock in the evening, as soon as the light faded from the day, Sasha would slink toward our bedroom, climb into his sanctuary of sheets and blankets, and lie there awake, with his knees to his chin.

I didn't know this was a pattern many Alzheimer victims follow. There is even a term for it: sundowning.

It would have been all right if Sasha had stayed in bed, but he didn't. After midnight he would suddenly become fully awake as if it were daylight, and he'd insist on getting dressed.

Sasha would wrestle with his clothes frantically, wrapping his jacket around his legs, tugging at the pants as he tried to pull them over his head.

"What are you doing?" I'd say.

"I have to go."

"Where are you going?"

"You don't understand. I have to go. I have to go."

He was too unpredictable to be left alone, so I would have to shake myself awake, follow him as he wandered around the house until I could persuade him to return to bed. Night after night his wandering broke my sleep and almost broke my spirit.

Sasha was on medication that couldn't be mixed with sleeping pills. I'd call the doctor and complain, "John, it's terrible. He doesn't sleep nights."

"Up the dose, Anne," he'd suggest. "Up the dose." It became the doctor's standard reply, along with the comment, "You have just got to face it. You're going to have to put him in some nursing home."

By now Sasha was also incontinent. He no longer had the capacity to respond to the signal he had to go to the bathroom. He went wherever he was, whether it was in our bed, or in his pants walking around the house.

I still shared the same bed with Sasha. I bought quilted pads, which are used in hospitals for patients. I tried to persuade Sasha to wear such a pad. I'd put it on. He'd tear it off.

The rubber pads I put on the bed only helped a little. I had to change the sheets so many times during the night that in the morning there was always a pile of dirty linen on the floor. Sometimes, exhausted, I'd steal into our guest room to try and get some sleep. Sasha invariably woke up. He'd switch on the light in the guest room and glare at my form under the blankets. "So that's how you feel about me," he'd say bitterly.

Instead of ignoring him, I'd feel guilty that I'd left him. I'd crawl back into our bedroom, and whether the bed was wet or not, I'd curl my body against his back, and comfort myself in the memory of how it used to be.

During the day my floors were a carpet of newspapers, laid out as if for a pet that wasn't housebroken. The sight of them littered throughout the house mutilated my last pretense at preserving normalcy. It seemed implausible that a man who had been so instinctively decorous in nature, could be reduced to such an undignified level.

There's a saying, "Where there's no solution, there's no problem." I knew I had to accept the unacceptable.

When I could no longer keep Sasha busy doing useful chores in the house, I concocted other ways to use up his time while I was at work.

I bought crayons, and a drawing pad. "Honey, do you see this tree?" I said to Sasha, leading him to the kitchen window that looked onto our garden. "Do you like this tree?"

"I love it," said Sasha simply.

"Would you do me a favor? Would you draw me a picture of this tree?"

"This one, or that one?" questioned Sasha, pointing to another tree at the back of the garden.

"This one, the closest one."

"All right."

I'd telephone him several times during the day. "Did you finish the drawing of the tree yet?" I'd ask.

"It's almost finished." It took him hours to complete one picture.

Our conversations were reduced to this pathetic drivel: I was the patronizing adult, Sasha the retarded patient.

The next day I'd choose something else for him to draw. "Sweetheart, can you draw this vase?"

At night, he'd show me his labored crayon creations. Occasionally, the object in the picture would be recognizable, but at other times the lines and colors collided across the page, the drawing a frenzied image of his mind.

I also took Sasha to senior centers, thinking it would help him to be with other people a few hours a day, but he'd look around the center for a few minutes, and abruptly decide, "You want to stay here—then you stay. I'm leaving."

I tried all sorts of places, all types of resources, but Sasha wouldn't—and couldn't—participate in programs. Eventually I hired sitters. I told Sasha I needed somebody to help me with the cleaning, because that was the only way he would allow anybody in our house, but invariably he'd telephone me at work, his fickle brain choosing this time to make a sane judgment. "She's lazy. She's not cleaning anything."

Unfortunately, he thought nothing of grabbing the woman by the hand, ordering her, "Here, you do this." I went through five women rapidly. One woman I hired rushed into my office, and dramatically rolled up her sleeve.

"See these black and blue marks," she shrieked. "This is what your husband did to me."

Sasha had become not just difficult to deal with, but potentially dangerous.

The only time Sasha physically threatened me was one night when Mary was in our house. Mary Lins was one of my closest friends, a woman I had known for many years, long before Sasha became ill. She was an assistant school principal, and she also volunteered her time as a librarian at the hospital where I worked. Mary was a tireless volunteer, a workaholic, the type of person who gives to everybody. Most of all she gave to me at a time when I needed to take.

Whereas most of my friends withdrew from my life after Sasha became ill, Mary used the illness as an invitation to strengthen our friendship. She became my confidant, listening for hours to all my troubles. She often stayed overnight at my house because she was concerned about me being alone with Sasha.

One evening Sasha had gone to bed as usual at six o'clock, and Mary and I were talking in the TV room. Sasha woke up and came to the doorway dressed only in his pajamas. The material of the pajamas was so thin you could see through it.

"Put your dressing gown on, Sasha," I said, embarrassed that he should appear this way in front of Mary.

Sasha ignored me. Lights startled him at night, and his expression was troubled.

"What's this woman doing in our house?" he demanded, pointing at Mary.

"Honey, it's our friend. You know Mary."

"What's she doing here? Doesn't she have a home?"

"She's staying the night. It's all right. Now why don't you go back to bed?"

"Get her out," said Sasha, his voice now raised. "She's a whore!"

"Sasha!" My voice rose above his. "Sasha, what are you saying?" I went toward him, but he met me halfway and gripped my arm, physically forcing me out of the room.

"Let's talk," I said, driving myself to sound calm. "Mary is our friend. You love her, don't you remember?"

"She's a whore," he shouted again. "If you don't tell her to get out, I'll throw her out." I stood facing my husband in the hall, fearful he might actually manhandle Mary. Was Sasha jealous of me spending time with my friend, or was his distorted mind spinning sick visions?

Mary joined us in the hall. "I'll go home if you want, Anne," she said softly.

"That's ridiculous." I took charge again. "There's no need for you to go anywhere."

Mary retired to the guest room and I led Sasha to our bed. I lay down with him, fuming silently, my anger once again too big to express.

In the morning Sasha entered the kitchen and said hello to Mary as if nothing had happened. My anger hadn't gone away. Usually I didn't harp on the things Sasha did, but this time I wanted to shame him.

"Do you know what happened last night?"

"No," he said. All innocence.

"You called Mary a whore to her face and tried to throw her out of the house."

"I couldn't have done that."

"You did."

"I must have been mad."

"Yes, you must have been." We were all going mad. "Aren't you going to say you're sorry to Mary?"

My husband, who only knew he had done something wretched because I told him he had done it, squirmed like a naughty two-year-old.

"Mary, please forgive me."

Mary forgave him. I didn't—not for a long time.

Later, Mary said to me, "Anne, I'm worried about you. I don't think Sasha would hurt you intentionally, but supposing he pushed you, and you fell down the stairs. He's becoming more irrational."

"It's not that bad," I maintained.

"It is, and you know it. You can't hide from the problem any longer. You've got to make a decision," insisted Mary, "and there's only one possible decision you can make."

In the middle of all this my mother died. I answered the telephone early one morning and heard a nurse tell me they had used shock treatment on my mother's heart. The rest of what she said didn't make sense, because the nurse littered her report with medical terms. At first I thought she was asking my permission to go ahead with some other treatment to help my mother. It took several minutes before I realized what she was saying.

I started to scream. Mary tried to pacify me. Sasha, who didn't understand what was the matter, put his arms around me and wouldn't let go.

I kept screaming. A mother is forever. You can yell at her, get annoyed with her, and kiss her. She is supposed to be always there. I screamed and screamed.

After a while, I called the hospital back. "Don't move her," I told them. "I want to see her."

My mother's face looked beautiful. I saw in her all the love she had ever given me, expressed and unexpressed. My own love was so intense it erased all traces of conflict that had existed between us. I felt if I touched her she would smile at me, but when I reached out all I experienced was death's coldness. Sasha and I stayed by my mother's side until they asked us to leave.

By this time I knew I would have to place Sasha in a nursing home. And yet . . . I clung to the thought that somehow I could delay the offensive act of turning Sasha out of his own home. I couldn't make such an irrevocable decision until I had explored every avenue. I kept hoping for a miracle. For a brief moment I thought I had found one.

I heard of a new health service program that was offering in-home health care for patients with acute problems. They had dependable "homemakers" who would come to the house to care for the patient, and Medicare was going to pick up the tab. I called immediately.

A woman from the project came to interview us. She was in her early twenties, a woman with a sweet smile, but her mind carried a clipboard of hardened questions.

She aimed the questions at Sasha. There was no way he could supply the answers, so I became his voice although she kept looking at him.

The questions continued for two hours, and all the time my hope kept building.

Finally, she turned to me and said, "There's no doubt he's eligible for our project."

My hope bounced up to the ceiling and beyond.

"You must realize," she added, "that even though he's obviously eligible we have two possibilities."

"Two? What are they?"

There was a research side to their project, she explained. They wanted to document the gaps in the present care available to the community. To accomplish this there would be a "control group" in their study; certain people would be denied the new services so they could be compared with those who received the special care. A "randomization process" would decide whether Sasha was one of the lucky ones chosen, or whether he would become part of the control group.

As she walked to the front door, I said, "How can I be sure Sasha is chosen for the in-home care?"

She shrugged her shoulders, the smile on her face not changing. She was gambling with my husband, running a lottery with human lives, but she acted as if there were nothing more at stake than a game of Bingo. Bingo, you might lose. Too bad.

"Can't you help us?" My tone stung with my disappointment. "I would do anything in the world to get this type of home care for Sasha."

The woman closed her briefcase. She lifted her head and drew out what she believed was a compliment.

"Your husband," she said, "is so fortunate to have you."

I thought: damn you!

We never heard from her again.

The first effort I made to find a nursing home for Sasha was done half-heartedly. I went through the motions almost in a trance. After work one day I visited the Jewish Home where I had placed my mother, and talked to the administrator to see if they had room for Sasha. I was told there were no openings.

On my way home it started raining. I had to make several changes by bus and I became soaked as I stood at each bus stop. The closer I got to home the guiltier I felt that I had even considered placing my husband in a home.

Sasha and his sitter met me at the door. "Look at you," said Sasha. "You are soaked through. You'll catch a cold."

He helped me remove my coat and shoes. His actions startled me. Once again his mind seemed clear; he was reacting normally to his wife's well being.

I went upstairs. A few minutes later Sasha followed me. He had my slippers in his hand. He had warmed them in front of the radiator.

"Here, put them on," he urged.

"Don't do this to me," I yelled at him. "For God's sake don't do this!" His mind was calm. My mind was unhinged. "I don't want you to treat me like an old woman. I don't want you to be my servant. Leave me alone."

The guilt engulfed me: I was being loved and cared for by the man I was thinking of turning out of our house. Without a word Sasha went downstairs. He looked as if I had beaten him. I sat and cried and cried.

It was, however, inevitable.

The small things made the decision for me. The stove turned on, and the saucepans I found when I came home, boiled to crisp black. The cigars, still lit, that Sasha threw out of the window, landing in gardens next to wooden houses. I don't remember exactly when I made up my mind. Maybe it was after another sitter walked out on us. Or maybe it was in the middle of the night, after dropping one soiled sheet on top of another, my senses zinging from lack of sleep.

If you want to picture hell, this is one way. The soul is hurt daily when a person you love crumbles in front of you. The constant twenty-four-hour care Sasha needed, extending over not just months but years, ultimately took its toll. Too many parts of me were worn out—the worker, money-maker, wife, mother, nurse, maid. I challenge anybody to have enough emotional and physical stability to take on all these roles, along with the pain, suffering, and sacrificing, without one day hollering one's heart out: "That's it! No more!"

For Sasha's safety and my own mental health, I knew I had to find a home for him. I began to make telephone calls. Note pads became filled with names of places recommended to me.

I took a day off from work. I made the first phone call at 8:30 A.M., and didn't stop dialing until night. One person referred me to another, one agency claimed another agency could help. By the afternoon I completed a circle; a person referred me back to the man I had spoken to at the beginning of my search. It was a rolling-stone effect. At the end of the day I had gathered nothing.

After weeks of telephoning, I realized I knew more about what was and wasn't available than the people in the agencies who were being paid to dispense such information.

Each facility had a different reason for not taking Sasha. The State Hospital, at that time, wouldn't take irreversible brain-damaged patients. Many nursing homes were filled, and had long waiting lists. Some said they couldn't handle "difficult-to-manage" patients. A couple noted I could only apply if I were on welfare. A few quoted incredibly high fees for nursing care.

I had no inkling it would be that difficult to place Sasha. My list whittled down to a few possible facilities. It was near Christmas, and Nicky was due home for the holidays. I decided I would postpone visiting these nursing homes until Nicky could come with me. It was a family crisis, and it was time for my son to participate.

Appropriately, it was during the Christmas season that an angel came into my life. Her name was Ratka. She was a nurse from Yugoslavia, who now worked in the United States with chronically ill patients and the elderly. As soon as she entered my house I knew she was different from every other woman I had hired to look after Sasha. To Ratka it wasn't just a job; she not only liked Sasha, she adored him. And Sasha, feeling her love, relaxed.

They shared a Slavic language so she understood him when he talked about his past, and when his stories became sentimental they cried together. She walked with him around our neighborhood, and took him on a bus. At home they sang Russian songs and danced to exhuberant Russian records. She made him move with life again.

Yet even Ratka noticed that every day the disease destroyed a little bit more of Sasha's brain. He was now deteriorating at a speed that was incomprehensible. Ratka only stayed with us ten days because she had a commitment to another family. She charged thirty-three dollars a day, which to me was a mountain of money, but she was worth every penny. For once I knew that when I left for work in the morning I didn't have to worry about Sasha. Ratka would make sure he was all right. When Sasha wanted to slip back into his routine of calling me a zillion times a day, she coaxed him away from the phone, allowing me a silence in my office I hadn't known for months.

If I had been able to find another Ratka maybe I could have kept Sasha at home longer, but there are only a few angels in this world who make house calls.

It was while Ratka was with me that I received an invitation to a ball celebrating the hundredth anniversary of Children's Hospital.

"This should be a marvellous event," I said to Ratka, showing her the invitation. "I've worked for this hospital for years. I feel close to so many of the people there. I wish I could go."

"What's stopping you?" questioned Ratka. "It would be a shame if you didn't attend."

"I can't even think about it. It's impossible."

"Of course it's not impossible."

"How can I go?" I flung my hand out in the direction of the newspapers lying all over the floor, waiting for my husband to make another mistake. Those newspapers symbolized the foulness of the disease and my life.

"How can you *not* go?" retorted Ratka. "You can't keep living like this. You've got to get out of this house more, and not just for work, but for fun. You have to do something for yourself, Anne," she said, quietly but adamantly. "Why don't you buy yourself a glamorous evening dress and go to that ball?"

I needed a Ratka to give me permission. More encouragement came from a physician friend, Dr. Petter Lindstrom, who invited me to join him and his wife at the ball. I accepted.

The Lindstroms picked me up at my home, told me I looked lovely, and pretended not to notice I was as skittish as a teenager facing her first dance.

Festive baskets of balloons paved the ballroom's edges. All around me were couples. I was in Noah's Ark, far too conscious I had left my mate behind. Then, as I stood with the Lindstroms, thinking I had made a mistake in coming, I heard somebody call my name. I turned to greet a friend . . . then another and another. The hospital's board members, the trustees, and many of the medical staff, all made their way toward me. They danced with me and propped me up. I wasn't allowed to be alone, or feel alone.

Early in the evening I met a man (I will call him George, although that is not his name), a lawyer with a beard and an impatient manner. George wasted no time in telling me that he was a widower and that his wife had died tragically several years earlier in a car accident.

I was polite and sympathetic, but I wondered why he was telling me these things.

When we got up to dance he asked me where my husband was.

"He's at home," I replied. "He has presenile dementia." It was the first time I had ever had the courage to say those words out loud. It seemed right somehow to match George's sad tale with my own.

"Good Lord!" was George's reaction. "I'm sorry."

"Well," I said, a little too flippantly, "poor George, poor Anne."

We danced a couple more times, and then I danced with others. For somebody who hadn't been to a party in years—who hadn't been out to dinner, or to a movie, or even socialized on a small scale since Sasha became so ill, this ball was dizzying. I floated with the balloons. Was this the real world? Would I ever return to such a carefree existence? I wanted the ball to go on forever.

"Can I take you home?" asked George, as he danced with me again later that evening.

"Thank you," I said. "I came with some friends, and I am sure they will be taking me back."

"They won't mind if you come with me," insisted George. "Please, it will be my pleasure to escort you."

I didn't want to make a fuss.

George's car was a convertible and since the night was warm he had the top down. Some stars appeared between clouds, and the Christmas lights flashed in the windows of the houses we passed.

While at the ball I had managed to forget my problems. It wasn't until George said, "Where do I turn to go to your home?" that I was jarred into remembering the hopeless situation waiting for me behind my front door. I told George to turn right on Twenty-second Avenue, and thought, "In a few minutes this marvelous evening will be over."

George's car stopped in front of my home. "It was nice meeting you," I said, turning to look at him. "I hope we'll be friends."

I had my hand on the divider between us, and George put his

hand on top of mine. "I hope we'll be more than friends," he replied.

He walked me to my front door. The porch light flooded our faces. George studied me in a way that made me feel self-conscious. "I'd like to have lunch with you tomorrow."

"I'm sorry. I can't see you."

"Why not?"

"I can't." I jabbered out my excuse: "It's my husband. I don't have anyone to leave him with."

"That's too bad." George shook my hand and left. I didn't call him back, but as I watched him get into his car, part of me went with him.

I had denied my sexual self for so long I was shaken when I found myself aroused by the thought of George. Initially, I hadn't considered him either handsome or intriguing, but in my imagination he grew into a knight. He could save me.

My life is a pattern of coincidences. George should have remained in my imagination, but within a few days I saw him again. I had just left my dentist's office when I noticed him coming toward me. His head was down, and his hands were pushed into his pockets. He hadn't seen me, so I stood in the middle of the sidewalk waiting for him.

"Oh no," he exclaimed as he raised his head. "Not you!" He kissed me on the cheek, and impulsively I said, "When you kiss a Russian woman, you have to kiss both sides."

He kissed the other cheek, and took my arm. "Where are you going?"

"I plan to catch a bus and go home."

"Let me drive you."

"No. There's no need."

"Don't be silly. Let me take you home."

As I got in his car, every part of me was alive. Before I realized what I was saying, or had time to understand what I was initiating, I said, "I have to tell you—you really send me." I used a colloqualism, a language that was foreign to me.

George took his attention away from the road and glanced at me. "What do you propose? An affair?"

"I don't have a name for it. This is just how I feel."

When we stopped at my house he said, "I'm going to be out of town for the next few days. I'll come and see you when I get back."

Chapter 6

ABANDONED

I telephoned Nicky at his college. I had warned Nicky in a letter that I was thinking of placing Sasha in a nursing home. Now I had to break the news to him he couldn't stay at the college in New York. Financially, I couldn't afford it, and emotionally, I couldn't do without him any longer.

"If you want to work, then it might be possible for you to go to college in California," I told him.

Nicky didn't sound upset about leaving New York. Over the telephone my son also accepted the idea his father needed professional care, and he promised to help me look for a suitable nursing home during his Christmas vacation.

Nicky hadn't been home for a year. On the day he returned to our house his smile quickly disappeared when he saw the condition his father was in.

"He's a skeleton, a ghost," said Nicky when we were alone. "Why didn't you tell me?"

Later, as he watched his father urinate in his pants, Nicky repeated, "I didn't think he was as bad as this."

To give me some rest, we began to take turns sleeping with Sasha. Nicky's energy quickly drained as he, too, tried to stop Sasha's senseless wandering during the night.

My son's concern for his father grew, as did his anger with
me. "You didn't prepare me," he said. "How do you expect me
to walk in and handle everything when I had no idea what was
going on?"

Nicky's anger, in many ways, was justified. While he was at
college, I had relayed a few details about Sasha, but had
concealed the grimness of our lives. I thought I was being kind.
Nicky had repeatedly groaned over the telephone and in his
letters about his own growing-up problems. I thought he had
enough to be concerned about without burdening him with the
size of my troubles. The mother in me worried: How could he
concentrate on his studies if he knew exactly what was
happening to his dad?

Besides, living with Sasha every day I wasn't fully aware of
the monstrous changes that had transpired in my husband
during the year that Nicky hadn't seen us. For me, the abnormal
had become normal. Nicky, on the other hand, stepped into the
middle of a mine that had already exploded, and was now
being asked to help salvage our remains. He was devastated by
what he saw.

Together we began to visit the few nursing homes that were
on my list. Not one was suitable, and most were terrible. There
was one place that was surrounded by barbed wire. A short
man with a sullen face unlocked the gate to let us in. It was like
entering a prison. Detached from the building that housed the
residents was a trailer for the staff. Outside the trailer was a
Cadillac.

The short man informed us he was the administrator. As soon
as we entered the building the stench stuck in our nostrils—the
unmistakable pungency of urine and human feces.

Every two or three years, television offers a shocking exposé
on the way we treat our elderly. From my sheltered living room
I had dismissed such exposés as media sensationalism. This
was undeniable: Men and women walking around naked.
Patients forgotten by the staff, hunched on bedpans. I saw men

urinating against doors, and even worse, I saw old people, too feeble to move without aid, leaning helplessly against walls, their feet in their own feces.

The newspapers in my home began to look good. At least I picked them up.

"This is disgusting," I said to the administrator. "How could you let them live like this?"

The man frowned. "That's the way these people behave," he said.

He went on to inform us it would be six hundred dollars a month for Sasha. We ignored him and walked out of the building. He hurried after us. "I could make it three hundred. You look like a nice lady."

When the gate closed behind us, I released my tears on my son's shoulders. Nicky, too, was having trouble holding back his emotions. "Mom, we'll never, never leave him in a place like this."

"It's all right honey," I sobbed. "We'll sell the house, we'll do anything. We'll find him the very best place, you'll see."

That particular home was state-licensed, and recommended to me by a social worker who was employed by the city. As soon as I reached my house, I telephoned the social worker and described the scene I had just witnessed. I thought he would be as outraged as I was at the conditions, but instead he replied, "These things bother you because you're not senile. It doesn't matter to them."

George was back in San Francisco. Nicky volunteered to stay home with his father if I wanted to go out. My son understood my wish to be with another man. Nicky had seen enough to know we had lost Sasha, just as surely as if we had lost him in death.

Years later I read a handbook for families dealing with dementias, published by Johns Hopkins University, which stated: "If a spouse is able to find a new relationship outside his marriage, no one is in a position to criticize that decision. Living and being loved is an important human need. Some people do build a new relationship at the same time that they provide loving care for the patient. Guilt feelings or blame from other relatives should be dealt with, with the help of a counselor if necessary."

I must admit that I didn't wallow in guilt. My need for George was strong enough to override everything. After all these years of not having a husband in the truest sense, I longed to be touched not only physically but psychically; I wanted someone to show me my life was worth living again.

George had telephoned me a few times while he was away and we had had long, surprisingly honest conversations. He was an articulate speaker, with an understated sense of humor that I found myself enjoying. His own laughter was loud and contagious.

When George arrived to pick me up I felt as if we had already developed a strong bond. He was my age, still had a healthy head of dark hair that was just turning gray, but his body was large and fleshy rather than muscular. He had told me he was considered a fat boy in his youth, and over the years he had always had to watch his weight. At the same time, though, he seemed lithe for such a big man. His grey-green eyes and the way he fixed his gaze on women reminded me of my father.

George took me to an expensive restaurant and ordered a fine imported wine after a drawn-out discussion with the waitress about wines, gourmet food, and her accent, which was Swedish. I later learned that George liked to engage waiters and waitresses in conversation, a habit that sometimes made me feel uncomfortable.

After dinner, George drove me to an isolated look-out point. He parked his car next to a van, and from our hilltop site I could see the moon reflected in the ocean.

"Aren't you afraid of parking here?" I said. "There have been a lot of rape stories in the papers lately."

To my embarrassment, George misunderstood me. He thought I was afraid he was going to rape me. "Nothing will happen to you that you don't want to happen," he said cryptically.

I was all nerves. "Isn't this where all the kids come?" I asked.

"Probably." George leaned back in the car seat and started to talk of other matters, but in the middle of one sentence he sat up slowly, and carefully unloosened his tie. It was a calculated move, utterly sexy. There was no doubt in my mind what he was about to do.

I had never been fondled in a car before. The forced close quarters enhanced my excitement. We didn't make love, but I did things I didn't expect of myself.

The next day George called and said it had been "sweet." As soon as he said those words I felt cheap. If only he could have said, "I love you," or "I care," but during all the time I knew George he was never able to soothe me with words. George added he was going away again, but would call.

The next few weeks Nicky and I spent all our time going from one nursing home to another. We saw a converted private house that rented out rooms to the elderly. The living room centered around the television, the electronic baby-sitter that kept the residents occupied. No other social activities were offered. In each bedroom there were two or three people, all of them ambulatory, and able to take care of themselves. They had to. The staff didn't do much for them.

The few places we liked wouldn't take Sasha. We were told that because of his unpredictable wandering he needed a structured program in a "locked facility." We discovered there were only two locked facilities in San Francisco and they were filled. Our search took us further and further away from our home, and I began to worry about how I would visit Sasha, since I had to depend on buses.

At first Nicky and I looked for a paradise, but when we found no such place existed, we settled for more earthly values: Were the patients clean? Did the place smell? Was there a sprinkler system? Was there a garden, somewhere for the patients to see the sun, stretch their bodies? We wanted to find a home where Sasha could exist, not just survive, a place that was more than a cell.

Eventually, we found a nursing home about forty-five miles away from our house. It was a modest, bleak building, but the rooms were decent, and the meals, although not exciting, were sufficient. The administrator appeared to know what she was doing, and told us she could handle somebody in Sasha's condition.

The evening before I took Sasha to the home I packed his suitcase. I was devoid of all feeling as I put his underclothes and his shirts in the case. The enormity of what I was doing numbed me. What do you choose to put into a suitcase that is never coming back? I picked up Sasha's best jacket. Do I pack it? Does it matter?

Throughout our marriage Sasha always told me, "You're so good to me." He used to say it with such warmth. He liked to acknowledge what I did for him, how much I cared for him. As I continued packing his clothes the phrase, "you're so good" kept tormenting me . . . yet I, who had been so good, was sending my husband away.

I hardly slept, knowing the suitcase was ready for the morning. As I felt Sasha's body next to mine I remembered all the years we had spent together, the physical and mental joining of two people.

To send him out of our bed, out of our house was horribly irrevocable. I couldn't pretend he might come back. Just as I had to finally accept there was no cure for Sasha's illness, I had to accept also this was a one-way trip.

To be responsible for somebody else's life is awesome because it's like playing God. It was devastating when I had to put my parents in a home. It can be devastating to part from a husband through death or a divorce. However, to part from a husband when he still needs you and you need him, and yet there is no way you can help each other, that is the worst. To take his life and put it away under lock and key, to play God with a husband . . . that is the very worst.

The next morning we all had breakfast. Nicky and I kept looking at each other—two edgy conspirators.

"You know it's for Pop's benefit," Nicky told me. He was also reassuring himself.

"He'll be safer there," I said emptily.

At age twenty-two, Nicky was experiencing the harshness of adult choices. His face carried the strain, for it wasn't any easier on him than it was on me to put Sasha in a home. Although he had been away at college during the last years there was no escape; the ultimate impact of seeing his father's brain shriveled had been violent to his soul.

"I'll get the suitcase," said Nicky.

We had heavily sedated Sasha, and Nicky had to help him into his Burberry coat. I was concerned it might be too much for Nicky to handle a car as well as his emotions, so I had asked Doris, our neighbor, to drive us to the home.

"Come on, the car's ready," called Doris, trying to be light-hearted so we wouldn't dissolve.

I sat in the front, and Nicky sat in the back with Sasha. As we got further away from the house Sasha began to fidget. He had a way of using gestures like words, and with a deliberate shrug of the shoulders he let it be known he wasn't sure where he was.

"It's okay," I said, pacifying him. "We're going for a ride in the country." Another unforgivable lie.

We drove across the Bay Bridge to the east side of San Francisco Bay. While crossing the bridge I looked at the sailboats below us and wondered what it must be like to sit in a sailboat and have nothing else to worry about other than the tides and the wind.

It seemed like an eternity before we got to the home. The

building had the appearance of a motel. There was nothing repulsive about the place, also nothing inviting. There were no flowers on the land, just bushes that didn't need upkeep, and a stretch of grass dotted with weeds.

Before we got out of the car I gave Sasha another doze of his tranquilizer. It was enough to keep him subdued.

His life was controlled by drops from a medicine bottle; mine was out of control as I led my husband of twenty-nine years into a lobby that reeked of disinfectant. I felt as though I were watching a surrealistic movie as a young man came forward to take my husband from me. I guess I expected some sympathy, some touch of human acknowledgment of the horror of what was being done, but they came with rigid faces and took Sasha away as easily as they took the suitcase.

Sasha was so sedated he didn't look back at us, as he was guided down the corridor studded with sprinklers into one of the rooms. I went into an office to sign the papers. How do you sign away a husband? I couldn't believe what I was doing. All along I had hoped there was another solution, and I still feel there has to be another way. If I could have found the type of professional help I needed I would have kept Sasha at home. I would have done anything to have not done what I was doing then.

Nicky and I stopped in the doorway of Sasha's room before we left. He was sitting on a bed talking to an aide. The dulled white walls of the room had only one nondescript print. For safety reasons, the small window was locked, there were no mirrors, and we had been asked to hand over any matches or cigarette lighters. If Sasha wanted to smoke one of his cigars he had to ask for a light; another chip of dignity dissipated.

Sasha didn't see us, and we didn't say anything. Besides, there was nothing we could have said that would have made sense either to him or to us. It was only after we got in the car and started driving away we allowed ourselves to feel. Then Nicky and I both wept, gripping each other tightly.

I cried for Sasha, and I cried for myself. I had enormous fears about being left alone without him, which was paradoxical; the illness had already taken him away from me.

This is the contradictory nature of the disease: Because you are left with a breathing body there is no conventional time of mourning. On one hand I had been grieving my loss for years, and conversely I had also been thankful Sasha was still in our house.

While he lived with me, I had a remnant of a husband. Now even that was gone. I was scared. I felt the loss as deeply as if I had become a widow. Yet, in all honesty, at the same time I also experienced another sensation that was undeniable—relief. I felt intense relief.

For once, I knew Sasha was safe. I thought: He's all right. I'm all right. And suddenly I was also aware that although I was still responsible for Sasha, I was no longer the prisoner of his disease. I was *free*. For years my life had shut down at sunset when Sasha went to bed. I hadn't been able to socialize, or lead any kind of normal existence. The sickness had isolated me from others.

It struck me: I could at last go out. I could visit friends. I was free!

Then came the guilt. How wicked of me to delight in my own freedom when Sasha's freedom had been taken away from him. God, I felt guilty. Within the next few hours I went through all the emotions in the book. Feelings somersaulted within me— heavy-heartedness because Sasha was no longer with me, light-headedness because my own life would have a chance again.

Appropriately, some friends, appreciating my need to contact the world again, invited Nicky and me to their home for dinner that night. During the meal they comforted me by saying, "Anne, you should have done it sooner. You waited too long."

Stressed the wife, "It was too much for you to keep working and looking after Sasha. I don't know how you did it all those years. He'll be much better off in the nursing home."

They tried to convince me, and I continued to convince myself. The wine went down, fusing the sorrow with the euphoria.

Around ten P.M. our friends came back to our house. They lingered there knowing it would be hard for Nicky and me to be left alone. We had managed to change the conversation to a light subject when the telephone rang.

It was the owner of the nursing home where I had placed Sasha. Her voice was loud, angry. "A member of my staff has just called to let me know your husband has become violent," she exclaimed. "You will have to remove him immediately."

"What do you mean?" I questioned. I felt instantly cold.

"He can't stay at the home. He's upsetting everybody. I'm going to lose all of my other clients."

"I don't understand," I fumbled. "You told me that your nursing home could handle my husband."

"Remove him immediately or else," she threatened. "He's destroying the place."

I tried to reason with the woman. "But my son and I came to see you beforehand and we explained what he was like. You said you had other cases like this, and you knew what to do." Panic was coming into my own voice.

"I never said anything like that," she retorted. "You lied to me about the condition of your husband. If you don't remove him this evening you'll be responsible for all the damage he has done."

"I can't come tonight. I don't have a car. I don't drive."

There was silence. I thought for a moment she was going to suggest I meet her the next day to discuss the situation, but instead she replied, "I'm calling from my house in San Francisco. We don't live too far away from you. My husband and I will come and pick you up tonight and take you to the nursing home."

We quickly got ready. Our friends left, shaken by the change of events. I didn't ask them to stay, for there are moments when friends can't enter the circle of a crisis. The problem was mine alone, and oddly I felt then—as I did through all the other crises that followed—that I was outside myself watching some passive flesh go through the necessary actions. The body, it seems, has its own way of anesthetizing itself against too much anguish.

The situation with Sasha had sounded so urgent we expected the owner of the home to arrive right away, but Nicky and I waited nearly two hours. Around midnight she drove up with her husband in a big Oldsmobile. Tired, we slumped down in the back of the car.

For most of the journey the couple ignored us, and when I finally said to her, "What am I supposed to do? Where can I take him?" she only answered, "Don't worry, I'll tell you."

Don't worry. Of course I was worrying. As the car moved past homes where families slept with uninterrupted dreams, I told myself I couldn't bring Sasha back to the house and go through the whole experience of having to turn him out again; you just cannot live the same tragic scene more than once. We had gone so far. There was no turning back.

As soon as we arrived at the nursing home the owner, still ignoring us, rushed out of the car to see her staff. They huddled together, their voices glaringly loud for the middle of the night. Nicky and I stood by feeling limp, helpless.

From what we overheard we gathered Sasha had taken a chair and tried to break it against a wall. My poor, darling Sasha. I could only guess his state of mind when he realized he was in a strange place, surrounded by unfamiliar faces. His confusion must have turned into rage.

And as I stood in the dark, waiting to find out what they were going to do with my husband, I, too, felt rage. There was anger because we had been misled into believing they would take care of Sasha. There was anger because we were made to feel like dirt that needed to be cleaned out. I was furious—and defeated.

Eventually they took us to see Sasha, who was lying, deeply drugged, and half undressed, on top of the bed. I packed his suitcase, this time just tossing things in carelessly. Then Nicky wrapped a coat around Sasha and carried him, still sleeping, out to the car . . . a son cradling a father, roles pathetically reversed.

"I can't take him to our house," I repeated to the owner. "What are we going to do with him at this time of night?"

"We'll go to Langley Porter," responded the woman. That's all she said, as we drove off.

My knowledge of the Langley Porter Institute in San Francisco was limited. I was aware it was for mentally disturbed patients, but at that time I had outmoded ideas about how people treat insanity. I pictured a place with padded cells, and the idea of putting Sasha into such a facility terrified me. I was still trying to make up my mind how to handle this whole situation when the car stopped.

"We're here," said the woman.

It was about two o'clock in the morning. I looked out the car window and saw the Langley Porter Institute smothered in a web of scaffolding. The building was being remodeled, and everywhere we looked there were barricades. The area appeared almost eerie, with only the fog moving under the streetlights.

We got out of the car. Sasha's drugs hadn't worn off so he leaned sluggishly against me. As I turned to ask the woman and her husband what we should do, I heard their car engine start up. I thought for a moment they were going to park, that they would come back for us. I couldn't believe they would just abandon us.

They did.

Later, I discovered they hadn't even tried to notify Langley Porter we were coming. Supporting Sasha between us, Nicky and I walked up to the Institute's heavy wooden front door, which was covered with steel. In the center of the door was a glass peephole. I peered through it and banged on the glass.

The door finally opened slightly. "What's the matter? What do you want?" said an unfriendly voice.

"Please, please help us." I talked faster than I had ever talked, as if each crucial minute decided our fate.

"I'm not sure if we can accept your husband," said the male aide after listening to my story. He left us in the gray painted hallway as he went to find one of the doctors.

A young man came out to greet us. When I saw him I was instantly dismayed. He looked younger than Nicky. How could he possibly understand what we had been through?

The young doctor extended his hand. As I shook it I saw his eyes. I felt instantly calm. They were the eyes of a man who had seen more in his life than I would probably ever know. He exuded such wisdom that just being near him made me feel safe.

"Why don't you sit here," suggested the doctor, "and I'll talk to your husband for a little while."

They returned about fifteen minutes later. "Obviously your husband needs care," the doctor concluded. Then he went on to explain that their Crisis Intervention Unit at Langley Porter offered brief hospitalization for patients, but this was not appropriate for Sasha because he needed a long-term facility.

"What am I to do?" I asked.

"We can keep him for a couple of days, and in the meantime perhaps our social worker can help you find another nursing home."

The next day I visited Sasha. He was engrossed in a conversation with an aide, and hardly noticed me. They were laughing, and my anxiety lifted. Maybe Sasha would adapt, after all, to new surroundings.

The social worker at Langley Porter informed me she had found one place that would take Sasha. I had also tried to find another home, but had met with no luck, so I seized her suggestion eagerly.

They sent him by ambulance to the new place. I didn't go with him, because I had to work. Somehow I had to keep making money to pay all the medical bills.

Four hours after Sasha was admitted, I got a call at my office. The woman on the other end of the line was upset. Her protests were all too familiar. Sasha, she said, had become physically aggressive with her staff. He had attacked a nurse, and twisted her arm. They were thinking of suing me, she added.

"S-suing me?" I stammered. "You're supposed to know how to take care of people like Sasha."

"We didn't realize he was this bad. You misled us." It was the same excuse I had heard from the home where we had first taken Sasha, and yet I had been painstakingly honest with each nursing home administrator.

"There is no way we can keep him here," continued the woman. "He has to be moved at once. You should take him to a psychiatric hospital. That's the only place for him."

"He has a physical illness, not a mental illness." It was my turn to protest.

"I'm sorry. In my opinion that's your only solution."

The situation was absurd. Within a few days my husband had been thrown out of two nursing homes, was only allowed to stay briefly at a psychiatric institute, and I was now being advised to send him to a psychiatric hospital. The doctors had told me senile dementia was a *physical* organic dysfunction. Surely society had a place for such people? Yet I had exhausted all the names in the yellow pages. I had run out of time and recommendations.

Sasha was moved to a psychiatric hospital.

It was around this time that an attorney advised me to set up a conservatorship over Sasha and his estate. This conservatorship, he told me, would allow me to sign contracts, sell our property if necessary, and manage all of Sasha's financial and legal affairs.

Sasha had signed a paper to voluntarily admit himself to the psychiatric hospital, but I knew he really didn't understand what he was doing. There is a law in California (the Lanterman-Petris-Short Act) that protects patients from being held in a locked facility against their will for an extended period of time, unless a court has established that the patient is a danger to others, or to himself or herself, or gravely disabled and is unwilling and incapable of accepting treatment voluntarily. Because of Sasha's deteriorating condition a court hearing was held that determined that Sasha was incapable of making these decisions voluntarily, and therefore could be placed involuntarily. It was a legal procedure that I had to go through so I could control a man who had become uncontrollable.

Morning after morning I woke up and entered a territory where the struggle was always the same. My hand would slide and find empty spaces in the bed where Sasha had been. My mind would sink, dreading its full conscious state, but my heart would act as if I had been running. What is it? I'm about to face something I don't like.

It snaps. Sasha has gone, but where has he gone? To a nursing home? Langley Porter? The home where he hurt the nurse? The psychiatric hospital? For a few seconds my mind stumbles, not wanting to know.

Then I wake up and cry. I'm alone.

Chapter 7

GRASS-ROOTS

I never stopped making the telephone calls. I followed even the flimsiest lead. If I thought some person or some place could help Sasha I called.

During my search I heard of a psychiatrist whose specialty was geriatric cases. I picked up the phone and dialed. He listened silently as I explained how Sasha had been turned out of three places in a matter of days. Seeking advice and empathy I said, "How can we treat sick people like this? There must be a suitable home for people with senile dementia. How can we allow families to go through such trauma?"

I expected to receive comforting words, but when the psychiatrist finally spoke all I heard from him was annoyance. Annoyance I had bothered him. Annoyance because he couldn't deal with me, or my husband, or my questions. His voice turned on me and said, "Mrs. Bashkiroff, you must realize society is not prepared for problems such as yours."

When I put down the receiver it was I who was annoyed. From his smug haven this psychiatrist had closed all doors, padlocked them, and told me there was no key.

The fighter in me wouldn't accept this to be the end. Doctors had said there was no cure for Sasha's disease. Social workers

had told me over and over again there was no facility that
would take my husband, but this psychiatrist had gone so far as
to tell me that society—our big, complex, caring society—
wasn't prepared to handle these problems.

My energy roared against this negativity. Damn it, I thought,
society had better be prepared to deal with us! I wasn't sure
how I was going to do it, but I knew I had to find a solution not
only for Sasha, but for all families who faced my situation.

Society was definitely going to be prepared.

When I first started trying to find a facility for Sasha, I
contacted the Jewish Home for the Aged where I had placed my
mother. I had hoped they would also take Sasha, but was told
the waiting list was so long it would take years before there was
an available space.

Then something bizarre happened. Sasha had been at the
psychiatric hospital for about a week when I received a
telephone call from a man who identified himself as an
administrator for the Jewish Home. "I'm calling from the
airport," he said. "I'm about to fly to Washington, so I can't
speak for long. Why didn't you turn up yesterday?"

"I don't knew what you're talking about," I replied, per-
plexed.

"We were expecting you to bring your husband to the Jewish
Home yesterday. Where is he?"

"I don't understand." I was even more puzzled. "I applied to
your home months ago, but was told there were no openings."

"We have room for him," stated the man matter-of-factly, but
before I could ask any questions he said, "I have to go. Call my
office and they'll help you."

I called the office and they verified they were indeed
expecting my husband. I welcomed my good fortune and didn't
probe further. To this day, I don't know who arranged for Sasha
to be placed in the Jewish Home, but I suspect a Jewish board

member of the hospital where I worked pulled some influential strings. I'll always be grateful to this anonymous friend.

The next day we moved Sasha from the psychiatric hospital to the Jewish Home for the Aged. Nicky and I went to the hospital to sign the papers for Sasha's release. The aides had dressed him as best as they could in his suit, and on the bed was the small suitcase that had followed him from place to place.

As we were leaving Nicky took out of his pocket a gold key chain that belonged to Sasha. "Here, Pop, I've been taking care of your keys for you," said Nicky. He put them in his dad's hand. "I thought you might like to have them once again."

Nicky's intention was to be kind, but neither of us perceived the importance of those keys to Sasha. His response was instantaneous. Usually when we spoke to him his face remained disturbingly blank; we never knew if our words registered in his brain, but on this afternoon he responded like a firecracker that had been lit. Sasha ran to the locked door of the psychiatric ward and tried to insert the keys.

His action was violent and cunning. He wanted to outwit us. He wanted out. Oh my Lord, I thought, he did know he was in a locked ward.

How much was he suffering, and what else went on in his dying mind?

The care at the Jewish Home was excellent. It was the only facility he'd been in that offered a semblance of home life. Sasha had a private room and we were allowed to thumb-tack family photographs on the wall. He even had his own toilet facilities.

The atmosphere was genial, and the nurses took time to talk to him. The Jewish Home restored Sasha's dignity but they, too, only kept him for a short time. It was not a locked facility and they weren't able to handle Sasha's unpredictable behavior. Sasha would walk from floor to floor, in and out of all the rooms, and if he saw somebody in bed he'd lift them up and try

and put them in a chair. He frightened the residents, as well as
the staff.

On three occasions he escaped. I'd get a call, always at night
around ten or eleven, from a frantic aide saying he was missing.

I'd imagine Sasha's confusion as he wandered down un-
known streets, shuffling along in his moccasins; he couldn't
wear shoes any more because his feet were now swollen from
edema. I used to see pictures of Siberian prisoners, their feet
protected only by wads of swaddling cloth, and in my mind's
eye Sasha, too, had become such a prisoner.

Each time, the police found him three or four miles away
from the home. Sasha still had the strength to walk long
distances. His strength was the last thing to go, and in many
ways it was his worst enemy because it made it difficult to
restrain him.

The psychiatrist in charge of Sasha at the Jewish Home made
a point of telling me it was against his medical ethics to
increase Sasha's medication to subdue him. A few days later he
called again: Since they couldn't subdue him, he said, I'd have
to move Sasha, preferably to a locked facility.

I appealed to the psychiatrist, but he refused to keep Sasha
any longer. Now, years later, I still question his decision to turn
Sasha out of this nursing home. His ethics said it wasn't nice to
overtranquilize somebody. My ethics said it wasn't nice to
throw somebody out of a good facility, especially since I still
hadn't found anything suitable for Sasha, except a psychiatric
ward. What if they had tranquilized Sasha just enough so he
could have adapted to the home?

Or was that unrealistic?

George called and asked if we could meet. I suggested he
come to my house, knowing full well I was not just inviting him
into my living room but also into my bed. I had been a married
woman for twenty-nine years, but I prepared for his visit with
all the excitement and romanticism of a young girl.

I went downtown and searched for appropriate bed linen. I wanted to lie on something different. I came home with navy butterflies scattered on white sheets. I also bought a Japanese-style housecoat, a Russian-gypsy record, and Cointreau.

When George arrived the butterflies were on my bed and also in my stomach. I served him coffee and Cointreau before the fire. We kissed and after a while I asked him if he wanted to go upstairs.

Once in my bedroom George began to take off his clothes. I remember thinking, soon he's going to be standing naked in front of me. I was still in my underwear. He came over, put his arms around me and released my bra.

It seemed simple and natural. It was the start of a relationship that lasted several years. Not all of our time together gave me as much pleasure as that one evening.

Sasha left the Jewish Home. Move number six. He returned to the psychiatric hospital where we had placed him before. I hated him being in that psychiatric ward. On one of our visits Nicky and I noticed Sasha had a black eye. The aides told us he had fallen, but we didn't believe them.

When Sasha was at the Jewish Home I paid nearly a thousand dollars a month for the medical and nursing-home bills. Although we had a comprehensive major-medical policy, our insurance did not cover these costs. The reason? Because Sasha's senile dementia couldn't be cured, his care was considered custodial in nature. "Custodial care" are the two time-bomb words for all patients who have brain disorders that can't be treated. It spells financial disaster. What we didn't fully understand until it happened to us, and what many people don't understand, is that insurance companies rarely cover custodial care. This has resulted in catastrophic financial problems for millions of Americans. Even Medicare, the health insurance program for the elderly, does not reimburse custodial care.

The only time our insurance picked up the bills was when

Sasha received active psychiatric care for his agressive behavior while he was in the psychiatric hospital. Insurance policies, however, will only cover treatment for psychiatric problems for a limited time (usually ninety days in one year), so even this financial relief was only temporary.

I knew that the psychiatric hospital was only a short-term solution for Sasha, and that soon I would have to find a long-term facility, which meant a return to custodial care and a return to paying thousands of dollars for housing him.

Sasha and I were middle-income Americans. We had some savings in the bank, some equity in our home, and I was earning a salary. Sasha was also receiving social security plus a small pension from his former company. We had too much money to be called medically indigent, and were unable to qualify for MediCal, the California program for the poor.

On the other hand, we weren't rich enough to survive the financial strain of massive extra bills over an extended period. The doctors had told me Sasha could live for years. I realized that before long I would run out of money. Eventually, I could lose everything we had worked for, everything we owned.

The conservatorship I had established over Sasha and his estate didn't solve my financial difficulties. Although I now had the legal right to manage Sasha's financial affairs and sell our home if I wished, everything we owned remained community property, and I was still responsible for all of Sasha's bills.

The conservatorship even cost me money. Periodically, I had to submit a detailed account of how much I had spent to the probate court for approval, and I had to pay for the court's costs, and all legal fees.

Some drastic steps to relieve my financial problems were suggested to me. "We can't help you until you qualify for welfare," one woman said. "If I were you I'd find a way get on welfare as quickly as you can."

A social worker told me, "Divorce your husband. If you don't divorce him, or hide your assets, the system will clean you out until you won't have a cent left. I see this happening to middle-income couples all the time."

Go on welfare? Divorce my husband? I couldn't believe people were offering these suggestions as viable solutions!

Later I learned that a divorce doesn't even necessarily help a spouse financially. For instance, in California there are two grounds for obtaining divorce or dissolution: irreconcilable differences or "incurable insanity." A severely brain-damaged person can be considered "insane" under the definition of the law, but dissolution due to incurable insanity *does not* automatically terminate the financial responsibilities of the former spouse.

Before Sasha and I emigrated to this country we had to promise we wouldn't be a burden to the American taxpayers. It was a promise we took seriously. For over twenty years we had worked in the United States, proud to be self-sufficient, contributing members of society. And yet now the same system dictated we couldn't get help unless we were destitute. It didn't make sense.

I didn't want to go on welfare. I didn't want the government to pay all my bills; forcing us both to become public burdens seemed a mockery of the system. In my opinion, it's not fiscally or morally sound to demand that both the patient and the well spouse exhaust all their money. This only results in two people having to go on welfare, rather than just the person who is ill. Wouldn't it be better to help families stay afloat so they didn't have to go on welfare?

To me, the solution was simple: I wanted to continue working and pay my fair share toward the care of my husband. All I needed was supplemental aid so I could keep up with the bills, and keep my self-respect.

I did get financial help, but not from the government.

Throughout Sasha's illness, my work at Children's Hospital was the glue that held me together. The thirty board members were all women and each of them, in her own way, gave me considerable emotional support.

They also assisted me financially, out of their own pockets. In my mail one day I found a letter from Nancy Lapham, a hospital board member.

"Dear Anne," it read.

"Everyone who knows you loves and admires you, and some of us who love you best would like to show this love in a more positive way.

"We know of all the problems you have had and in an effort to provide something a little more concrete than sympathy, we have accumulated a small amount of the stuff that makes the world go around.

"Enclosed is a check which you will receive monthly. The amount is not large, but we hope it will help.

"With xxxes from us."

It was signed by Nancy, and ten other members of the board.

Meanwhile, I was still a mother dealing with a son who had problems of his own. Nicky was having difficulty readjusting to life in California. He missed his New York college, and although he had been accepted at the University of California, Berkeley, he didn't know whether he should pursue his studies or go to work. He had lost contact with his former San Francisco friends and hadn't yet made new ones.

What's more, Nicky hadn't yet come to terms with his father's illness. Often, after visiting Sasha, my tears ran until my eyes became puffy, but Nicky's face remained stiff and dry. He once told me I cried enough for both of us, but it would have been so much healthier for him if he, too, could have shown emotion.

There was an incident that was particularly painful for Nicky. It happened while Sasha was at the Jewish Home. On one of our visits I went up to Sasha, greeted him with a kiss and then said, "Darling, look who is here. Nicky's here."

"Who?"

"Your son, Nicky."

Sasha had a benign smile. He turned and used it on Nicky, but his face held no recognition.

For a few seconds I stood awkwardly between father and son. Inanely I said, "Honey, don't you remember your son?"

I could hear Nicky panicking as he cried out, "Pop, don't. Pop, this is me. This is Nicky."

"No, how can it be?" replied Sasha, from a place years away. "When did you get to be so big?"

Soon after that Nicky stopped visiting his father.

Tragedies can bring families closer together, but the opposite also occurs. Our family was ripped apart. I started fighting with my son. Often we fought over his refusal to see Sasha. Nicky said he'd be willing to visit his dad if it helped in the slightest way, but he didn't think his presence made any difference. He argued there was no visible change on his father's face when he did see him; his father didn't know him, and wouldn't miss him. Nicky also said it hurt him to watch his dad's deterioration. I told Nicky it hurt me if he didn't see Sasha.

"Your father is sick," I said, pulling out the old guilt line, "and yet you don't have the decency to visit him. I need you to come with me. How can you be so selfish?"

I accused him of other terrible traits. I whipped him with my tongue, and Nicky in return was equally unkind to me.

My relationship with George didn't help my relationship with my son. What angered Nicky the most was that I used to ask him to leave the house when George came to visit. George never stayed overnight so Nicky knew I was just asking him to leave for a few hours. Since Nicky had been away at college I had enjoyed a certain freedom from my mother-role. I also thought Nicky had learned to be independent, but my twenty-two-year-old son complained he had no car, and nowhere to go. He interpreted my request to leave as "throwing him out of the house."

In the morning I'd tell Nicky, "George is coming tonight and

I'd like to be alone with him. Can you please make plans for the evening?"

During dinner I'd remind Nicky, "George will be here at eight. Have you made plans for the evening?"

There would be no response, but after dinner Nicky would move to the TV set. As the time for George's arrival grew closer, I'd get nervous and say, "Nicky, I'd like you to leave. George will be here soon."

Again, no response. Fifteen more minutes would go by. Then I'd demand: "Nicky, please go!"

This scene was repeated many times. Nicky would get up, glare, and slam every door he passed until he reached the front door. He'd slam that one too.

Nicky didn't object to my having a relationship with George. On the contrary, my son said he liked him, and at first he encouraged me to see him. Yet later, when he saw how preoccupied I was with the romance, he began to feel neglected.

I needed George. But Nicky needed me. I tried to explain to Nicky I had to recapture my feelings as a woman before I could continue my role as a mother. He tried to explain to me he had already lost his father and now he believed I, too, was abandoning him.

It was around this time I learned I had to have surgery. My doctor informed me I had a large tumor on my ovaries. There was a possibility, he said, it could be malignant.

I came home and prepared dinner. I waited until the end of the meal before I told Nicky, "I have to undergo surgery."

"When?" he said.

This was Friday. "Monday. I have to be in the hospital Sunday night."

I started to give him the details but before I could finish Nicky left the table and left the house.

During the evening the pain in my stomach intensified, and by the morning my doctor, whom I had called several times during the night, said, "It looks as if we'll have to operate immediately."

Nicky came home just in time to drive me to the hospital. Surgery went well, and the tumor was not malignant. I only stayed in the hospital for a few days. On my last night I was given a sleeping pill to make sure I slept soundly. Around two A.M. I awoke to find a flashlight aimed at my face, and the night nurse shaking me. "Mrs. Bashkiroff, your son is on the telephone," she said. "He said it is an emergency."

I picked up the phone and heard Nicky sobbing. One of our Russian records was playing in the background.

"Mom, Mom, I'm sorry, I'm sorry," he said, apologizing for waking me up.

"Honey, what's the matter?" He didn't make much sense, but I quickly grasped what was important: My son had at last broken the dam to his emotions. As I tried to calm him, I told the nurse to ask my neighbor, Doris Dunbar, to go to our home. I wrote down her telephone number, and gave it to the nurse. I talked to Nicky until I heard the doorbell and knew he was no longer alone.

"Anne, I have the answer to your problems." Nancy Lapham was on the telephone. "A friend of mine," she went on, "is a board member of the San Francisco Mental Health Association. She's been a volunteer with them for over fifteen years. She knows everything there is to know about mental health. Her name is Jane Ophuls. I spoke to Jane and told her about Sasha, and how many times he's been moved. She was appalled, but she's sure she can help you. You must call her."

I thanked Nancy and promised I'd contact Jane, but privately I thought it was futile. Too often I had heard somebody had the answer, and too often I had been disappointed. Nonetheless I called.

Jane Ophuls was sympathetic and reassuring. She said that

Barbara Cohen, a staff member of the Mental Health Association, knew of a nursing home that was tailor-made for Sasha.

Unfortunately it was another disappointment. When this nursing home heard about Sasha's behavior in other facilities they said they couldn't keep him either because he sounded too difficult.

Barbara and Jane weren't discouraged. They still thought it wouldn't be hard to find a facility for Sasha. Both women suspected that the only reason I hadn't located a good place was because I was a lay person and didn't know where to look.

As a black woman, a social worker, and program associate of the Mental Health Association, Barbara had paved her own shortcuts through the labyrinth of bureaucratic agencies. Using all her professional know-how Barbara investigated every source, checked every agency and every regulation.

She discovered what I had discovered; there was no suitable place in San Francisco or the nearby communities for my husband. And there was no agency or program that gave financial aid to middle-income families for long-term custodial care.

Barbara and Jane couldn't believe they had worked all these years helping people, and yet they couldn't help me. Jane presented my case to the Board of Directors of the San Francisco Mental Health Association. She was given the backing of the board to investigate my problem further.

By now, Sasha had been at the psychiatric hospital for nearly a month, but once again he was moved. His edema, caused by congestive heart failure, had become worse. The doctors decided to send him to a medical center for treatment. I was thrilled Sasha was leaving the psychiatric facility. I was glad his edema had become so bad he needed special attention. Imagine that! Imagine being glad your husband is sick enough to be hospitalized because you believe he will get better care at a medical center than at a psychiatric facility, or even most nursing homes. This was the craziness of my situation.

As it turned out the care Sasha received at the medical center was not as good as I had hoped. The nurses didn't have time to pamper Sasha. At mealtimes they delivered his food on a tray and left, but my poor Sasha didn't have the faintest idea what to do with food—whether to use a fork, a knife, eat it with his hands, or drink it. Whenever possible I tried to be with Sasha at dinnertime so I could feed him. I was concerned he was getting too thin.

Most of the time the nurses tied Sasha to a wheelchair. The ties were loose enough so he could move around, but strong enough so he couldn't get out. To see my husband bound in such a way disturbed me, but I also understood they couldn't allow him to wander aimlessly.

Sasha stayed at the hospital for twelve days. The whole time I worried about where I could move him next. Sasha had lived most of his life as an immigrant—a stateless man—until he had become a citizen of the United States. He had faith in American democracy, and yet in many ways his illness had made him less than stateless; he had become a nonperson, unwanted and uncared for by the American system he had cherished, and that he had believed would take care of him!

A hospital nurse and discharge planner gave me a list of nursing homes. Methodically, I went down the list, as I had done with so many other lists. I called each home, and Nicky and I visited a few. It was the same story; they wouldn't accept Sasha.

However, there was one difference with this list. It gave the names of places in other towns. When Barbara Cohen had tried to find a facility for Sasha she had only looked at local communities because she knew if the home was miles away I would have trouble visiting my husband. I now recognized I had to accept anything, so I called a place located in a town that was a two-hour drive from my house in San Francisco.

I rented a car and Nicky drove me to see it. Several cottages faced a large handsome courtyard, and encircling the cottages was a high wall. The wall made this a locked facility but what I immediately liked about the home was that the patients were allowed to move in and out of the cottages and around the courtyard. They weren't locked inside one building.

The place was too expensive, and too far away, but they said they could care for Sasha. I agreed to send him there.

It was move number eight. In three months Sasha had been moved eight times. While Sasha was still living with me I had often seen him confused but after these rapid moves he not only didn't know where he was, he didn't know who he was. His spirit had vanished along with his mind. Physically he hadn't died, but in every other way we had lost him.

I blame society. The fury I felt when I heard the psychiatrist say, "Mrs. Bashkiroff, you must realize society is not prepared for problems such as yours," was the same fury I experienced when I saw what these moves had done to Sasha. He had become what is disgustingly called a "vegetable."

This decay, I believe, could have been delayed if he had stayed in one place. Surely it is the responsibility of society to provide a safe, secure environment for people with Alzheimer's disease or other brain disorders. You wouldn't drag a man with a broken leg over a bumpy, rocky road, and yet a man with a confused mind was allowed to be dragged from one place to another.

As far as I'm concerned, our system destroyed what was left of my husband.

However, as a citizen of the United States I am also aware of this: The strength of our system lies in the freedom to make changes and choices. Where there is a wrong there are individuals who are willing to work and make things right.

Two of these individuals were Jane Ophuls and Barbara Cohen. They hadn't forgotten me. By this time I was committed to helping others, and Jane and Barbara also wanted to change the system that failed families such as mine.

"I'd like you to come with me to a meeting at your district community health center," said Jane one day, "and tell them about all the problems you've had with Sasha."

The meeting was a failure. When I finished my story they asked me a few questions, but they appeared antagonistic toward me. One woman, who owned a nursing home in San Francisco, even seemed insulted. Her home, she said, was a good home.

"It probably is," I replied, "but I needed a locked facility. You couldn't have handled my husband."

They didn't want to hear any more. They switched their minds to other business matters. I got up to leave. As I reached the door a man came towards me. "I want you to know that I was listening to you," he said. His face held compassion. "Something has to be done. Things can't remain the way they are."

The man's name was Peter Jamgochian, and many years later I met him again. "If it hadn't been for you, Peter," I told him then, "I wouldn't have made any other speeches. Your one outstretched hand made me feel all was not lost."

Jane invited me to another meeting, explaining this one was particularly important because it was a meeting of the Mental Health Association's Community Assessment Committee. Their job was to assess the mental health services in San Francisco, draw attention to inadequacies, and encourage new programs.

About fifteen people sat around an oblong table. Dorothy Gibson, a clinical social worker, chaired the meeting.

I sat next to Jane. I heard a psychiatrist talk about some problems he couldn't resolve, and I heard other people describe problems they couldn't resolve. I kept hearing how awful things were, and the more I heard this the angrier I felt. My spine became taut.

Here were the do-gooders doing what? How many meetings

had taken place, and how much time, energy, and money had been spent on these problems, all resulting in . . . nothing? I was exasperated by the apparent uselessness of it all.

"I want you to meet Anne Bashkiroff," Jane was saying. "She is here to tell you her personal story."

I pushed myself back from the table and began. I repeated everything I said at the first meeting, but this time my voice was stern and determined. I wasn't a woman begging for help. I was a woman *demanding* something be done. I wasn't crying out for myself. I was crying out for everyone who was suffering in our society.

When I finished there was silence. Their reaction made me think of leprosy; for months these professionals had listened to doctors describe hideous sores on bodies, but most of them had never actually seen the victims or understood the disease. Then I came along and said, "You want to see what leprosy is like. Here, take a look at me. I'm a leper."

They looked. And then everybody started talking.

As I listened my cynicism subsided. It became obvious these people hadn't gathered merely to complain and compare notes. They wanted to find solutions. True, they didn't yet know what to do, but they were eager to throw in advice and opinions.

What followed was a victory, not just for me, but for the American grass-roots system. The rest of the meeting was an untested recipe. We had a mix of people. We then took some ideas and facts, gave them a bit of juice, and kept stirring until something developed.

It was decided doctors needed to be educated about the problems brain-damaged victims and their families encounter. It was decided *everybody* needed to be educated. "Let's sponsor an educational conference as well as a press conference to bring the issues to the attention of the general community," suggested one person.

"Anne needs to be on that conference," said Thomatra Scott, a youth program coordinator with the Economic Opportunity

Council. Scotty, as he was called, was a black man who was known for his forthright manner and the black beret, boots, and dashiki that he always wore. "She needs to say what has happened to her," continued Scotty, "and then it will bring the other people out of the closet so they'll say, 'yes, it happened to me too.'"

I had my own ideas about what was needed. Cancer victims meet to support each other, I said, so why shouldn't families of brain-damaged victims get together?

"This is a must," I emphasized, "because when a family member is brain-damaged it really cuts your life into pieces in every way, and if you can talk it out with somebody it helps. Perhaps you've experienced something that they haven't. Perhaps they know something that you don't. It's just the feeling of you're not alone—you're all part of the same problem."

Dr. Carl Jonas, a psychiatrist, then spoke. He had observed the anger in my voice, and knew such anger ought to be directed. "I'm very much impressed by your report," he said, looking at me kindly, "and also your suggestion that you, along with other people who have gone through this kind of experience, need to find a way to meet one another. I'd like to propose that's the place to start. You're going to keep more up to date on what's available than any dumb card-index system at somebody's office. You know what's happening. You're dealing with it every day because of your spouse's involvement in it."

"In other words," interrupted Dorothy Gibson, the chairman, "she's the expert."

"That's right," asserted Carl. "Not only that but then you and your group have the basis for coming back to us and letting us know what we can do."

Sally Lewis, a public health worker, sounded timid when she asked her question, but in it was the seed of the future: "Could we sponsor an organization of concerned families, or something of this sort?"

"How do we identify these families?" questioned one woman.

Scotty spoke up again. "I would like to identify the resources first. We need to give some services to these people," he insisted, adding that they should investigate what resources were available to aid victims and their families. "What I'm saying is that the families don't have the time to do the investigating. What I'm saying is Anne has investigated until she damned nearly dropped. I'm saying we need to help her find some other avenues. This is heavy. This is very heavy action."

Scotty was challenging us.

I urged him and the others on. "I've done my suffering," I said, "I've done my crying. I've done everything. That's behind me. I'm looking ahead now. I want to do something positive."

From that meeting, at the suggestion of Dorothy Gibson, a task force was formed. We became the first organization in California to work for social and political change for all brain-damaged people.

Chapter 8

THE ACTIVIST

We called ourselves the Family Survival Task Force. Dorothy Gibson and I became founding members, along with John Bosshardt, an attorney; Barbara Cohen, who had helped me so much in the past; Suzanne Harris, vice-chairman of the Mental Health Association's Community Assessment Committee (Sue had a personal reason for belonging to our task force. Her husband had brain damage, caused by three cerebral hemorrhages); Gatha Hesselden, who became our first chairman; Dr. Carl Jonas; Sally Lewis; and Jane Ophuls, who remained our guiding light.

There were others who joined us later. We were a tenacious group, and with our varied backgrounds we were able to cross-fertilize skills. Each of us, in our own way, played an important part toward our success.

Publicity about our small group came quickly. Caroline Drewes, a feature writer with the San Francisco *Examiner*, wrote an article about my situation with Sasha. I didn't particularly like the idea that my personal life was now being exposed in newspapers, yet it was necessary. The social stigma of the disease had kept too many of us silent. I hoped that if I spoke out, perhaps others would also speak out.

Caroline's article had such an impact I was soon being interviewed for radio and TV. One day Barbara telephoned me at work and announced, "Anne, you have a chance this afternoon to appear on a talk show in front of a studio TV audience. Can you get off work? I'll pick you up and take you to the station."

What happened next was typical of TV land where deodorant commercials are squeezed between hard news stories of wars and rape. When we arrived at the station we discovered I was to follow a dog act. As I stood backstage I could hear the audience laughing at the dogs' antics. Believe me, it wasn't easy going on stage afterwards and trying to turn people's minds from a comical animal act to a discussion about a serious issue!

Each time I, or any of the task force members, received publicity, the letters poured in from people who told us that they, too, were having catastrophic financial and emotional problems caring for a brain-damaged member of their family. Too many of these letters sounded desperate, and as we read them we realized we were uncovering a major national tragedy.

Exact figures on the prevalence of brain damage in the United States are difficult to find, because there is no formal system for collecting nationwide statistics on noncontagious diseases. The National Institute of Neurological and Communicative Disorders and Stroke estimates "unofficially" that approximately twenty-two million Americans suffer from neurological and sensory disabilities. That is probably a low figure.

Consider, too, that the number of the nation's elderly will more than double by the year 2030, to the point where one in five Americans will be over sixty-five. Five to ten percent of these people will suffer from Alzheimer's disease.

If you mutiply these millions by the family members of brain-damaged victims who are also paying a social and economic price for the illness, then you are discussing a monumental crisis.

Our task force met frequently. I have always been proud that

Family Survival represented, right from the start, victims of all forms of brain disorders, no matter what the cause. Alzheimer's disease, Huntington's, Parkinson's, multiple sclerosis, brain tumors, stroke, head injuries . . . these are all kindred disorders that need similar services.

A couple of years after we formed our task force I read a government report by the "Commission for the Control of Huntington's Disease and Its Consequences," which stated, "The Commission believes that in an era of scarce resources and increasing demands, costly and redundant programs for individual diseases are no longer feasible. . . . The territorial behavior that sets one disease sufferer against another must give way to a united approach aimed at achieving compassionate care, treatment, and cure for all these diseases." This statement happened to reflect our viewpoint at Family Survival.

Our first goal was to organize a family support network to give each other advice and emotional courage. We also published a handbook outlining financial and legal alternatives for families. In addition, we shaped one other priority: It became our dream to win either state or federal legislation that would provide services and financial assistance for all brain-damaged adults. It was a matter of breaking new ground. No such legislation existed in any state.

Barbara Cohen and I began to visit legislators and their aides. In many ways I was naive. I thought if I simply told these politicians about our needs things would change overnight. It took longer than that.

Fortunately, there was one politician who did take an immediate interest in our cause. Barbara arranged for me to meet Assemblyman Art Agnos, a recognized advocate of humanitarian programs. I felt at ease with this man as soon as I saw him. His face and attitude were friendly, and his interest in my story seemed genuine.

Like so many people, Art Agnos wasn't aware of how

families were affected by chronic illness until I told him about my problems. After we met he conducted his own research into what services were available for brain-damaged adults and their families. It wasn't long before he, too, became convinced there was an unmet need that required attention.

Art Agnos began to work with us toward a full-blown legislative remedy.

As I began to express myself politically, a change took place in my personality. Throughout my married life Sasha had told me not to be inhibited, but it wasn't until I was on my own, when I had no choice but to take charge of my life, that I became more flamboyant, both in my speech and in my looks.

I had always gone to beauty parlors, had my nails done, and dressed well, but my taste in clothes had been toward the tailored look, in keeping with the office life I had led. Gradually, I began to choose clothes that were more feminine. I bought caftans, bright-colored dresses and scarves, and since I couldn't afford expensive gems I developed a good eye for exotic costume jewelry. After marrying Sasha I had returned to being a brunette, but now I let the hairdresser make my hair lighter and lighter until I once again became the blond I had been in Shanghai.

Although my outward appearance may have improved, the inside of me was still in turmoil.

My life was in fractions. Some aspects of my life felt good; my work with the Family Survival Task Force and my job at Children's Hospital challenged me and satisfied me. Yet the private part of my life was as distressing as ever. The pain of seeing my husband transformed into a torso never diminished. My spirit never left that darkness.

I lived in two worlds divided by a locked gate to a nursing home. When I approached that locked gate the reality of these two worlds tightened my stomach. I couldn't get used to the idea: Sasha's in there and I'm out here.

I couldn't get used to crossing a psychological as well as physical gate every time I saw my husband. I'd arrive, hoping to see a residual of the man I had married, but all I found was a strange stranger. On one visit I went up and offered a hug, until the man I was hugging made an unfamiliar utterance. With a shock, even revulsion, I withdrew. I was hugging the wrong person. In this ambience they had all begun to look alike, withered beings, their individuality defeated.

Sasha had become a man who put his dentures in his pocket, never in his mouth. A man who would smile his gummy smile at me because he knew I cared for him, but didn't know I was his wife. A man who no longer spoke Russian or English. He had returned to his childhood, to the ghost of his German governess; his words were now in German only. However, there was one small loving reminder of the past: He often kissed the hands of his nurses, the same way he had greeted all women in the past.

On another visit, while I was holding Sasha's hand, my fingers touched an alien smoothness. I looked down to find his wedding finger stripped. Over the years the wedding ring had wedged itself into the skin. It couldn't have slipped off, but I had no way of knowing whether he had given the ring away, or whether someone had taken it.

It was a four-hour round trip to see Sasha. I persuaded Nicky to come with me once, but he wouldn't go again. Because I couldn't drive, a friend occasionally took me to the nursing home. The rest of the trips were made with George; a lover taking me to see a husband I loved. My two worlds pieced together.

When George volunteered to drive me to see Sasha I regarded it as a gracious gesture, one of the kindest things he ever did for me. George knew I loved Sasha, and that I would never have considered seeing another man if Sasha had been well. Sasha's brain damage had left me in a difficult position. I'd lost my husband as permanently as if by death, although I couldn't claim windowhood because his body was still living. At the same time I had needs as a woman; I wanted—and needed—a man in my life who could return my love.

After twenty-nine years of marriage, love to me was as basic as bread. I was used to it being there all the time. My marriage to Sasha had gratified my very being. It was this type of love I hoped to have with George, but with George I was ready not just for love, but for a romance. When I first married Sasha I knew little about men. Now, as a mature woman, I was far more prepared to express ardor. For one thing, I was willing to experiment sexually—a side of me Sasha would have adored to see, but missed. I gave everything I could give to George, emotionally and sexually. I gave so much I assumed that he belonged to me. And that was the mistake I made. George resisted belonging to anybody.

When we were together George offered me solace, affection, and at times immense happiness, but he would only grant me so much and no more. I was never sure whether it was because he was afraid to risk a close relationship again after his wife's death, or whether it was just his nature to hold back. Perhaps it was a bit of both. On one level he was gregarious, easygoing, and was successful in his career. And on the other level he was inclined to be secretive, needed his privacy, and had few close friends.

When I told George I loved him he responded, "I wish you wouldn't say that."

"Why not?"

"I just don't like it."

"You must understand Russians are naturally demonstrative, "I said defensively. "I love you for now, for this minute . . . I love you."

George gave me a gift once, a whimsical fluffy toy dog, and on the card he wrote, "in appreciation." When I questioned him about his choice of words, his answer was a solemn explanation that, "Appreciation is more meaningful than love."

Eventually George was able to say, "I love you too," but I was aware that it was hard for him to label his emotions. To me, it was not only important to bring out the emotions, but also the soul—always the soul. There were evenings when I thought I had touched this unseen core of him; on these evenings as we lay before my fireplace, our conversation became as intimate as our love-making. Yet after an evening of such talk, he'd put on his jacket and walk out without telling me when I would see him again. Each time he left my house he left my life. He never said, "I'll call you." I never even knew *if* he would return.

However, George must have needed me as much as I needed him because he did keep seeing me. But it was an unstable relationship and soon after it began I sought the help of a psychologist; my thoughts were as muddled as my life.

Unfortunately, I wasn't as honest with the psychologist as I should have been. I dwelled on surface problems and as much as she probed I only allowed her to catch a slight glimpse of the deep shadows inside of me. As a result my sessions with her were of little benefit.

Our Family Survival Task Force, under the auspices of the San Francisco Mental Health Assocation, held its first public meeting on March 29, 1977, in the basement hall of a church.

We invited families and friends of brain-damaged adults, as well as professionals who worked with brain disorders. Although we had attracted a lot of publicity we weren't sure how many people would attend. We anticipated about fifty, but over two hundred people turned up.

Gatha Hesselden, our chairperson, gave the welcoming address, and Suzanne Harris briefly presented the goals of our Task Force. Suzanne spoke eloquently but it was a difficult speech for her; her husband, a victim of brain damage, had died two weeks earlier.

When I got up to talk I held my notes in my hand, but I didn't need them. I knew what to say. First I wanted the audience to know about our lives before Sasha's illness struck, and so I told them about meeting Sasha in Shanghai, and how he had followed me to America, marrying me two hours after he got off the ship.

"As time went on we had a son," I said, "and we thought the world was our oyster. We worked hard and we had a lot to show for it. In those days the dollar went further. Our boy attended private schools and we were a happy family. Moreover, we realized we not only had good jobs, but we had jobs that provided ample insurance coverage. We had double coverage. I had coverage on my side, and my husband had coverage on his side, so we thought nothing would go wrong if either of us became sick."

We were living, I stressed, with a false sense of security. Eventually, when Sasha did become ill our insurance coverage, which we had so much faith in, totally failed us.

"God forbid that an irreversible brain disorder should hit any of you," I continued, looking directly at the audience, "because if you are a middle-income family there is no public or private coverage, no federal support, no state support—nothing. You are on your own. So please be aware of this.

"I also want to point out that even though my husband was an older man, brain damage can happen to anybody. Brain damage can come about as a result of an accident, alcoholism, or aneurysm. There are many causes."

I wasn't going to let this audience off lightly. If they walked away from this conference thinking my problem was not their problem then we were all wasting our time.

In every audience you can find a few faces that give you boldness. These are the attentive faces; their thoughts are accessible in their eyes. I concentrated on these faces as I chronicled the eight moves Sasha made in three months.

"He is now in a locked facility in another town. It costs me nearly one thousand dollars a month for his care at this facility. Then, of course, there are the doctors' bills that Medicare does not cover, and the pharmaceutical costs Medicare does not cover, and a thousand and one other services you don't know whether your husband needs, but the sanitarium decides he needs it, and therefore he gets it, and you get the bill.

"I imagine most of us here consider ourselves to be middle-income families. I don't know how many of us could support paying one thousand, twelve hundred, or sixteen hundred dollars a month for years and years."

Besides discussing the economic disaster of long-term care for brain-damaged patients, I also talked about the lack of services for the patient and family, and the emotional pit these individuals fall into.

"Remember this statement," I commanded. "A psychiatrist said to me once, 'You must realize society is not prepared for a problem such as yours.'

"So what is the answer to that? Am I supposed to throw my husband off the Golden Gate Bridge? Am I supposed to jump off the Golden Gate Bridge. What is the answer to that?" I repeated.

"The problem of placing somebody in a facility is a terrible tear to the family," I went on. "I am alone. I'm not a wife. I'm not a widow. I don't belong in society anymore. My whole life is broken up. One has friends, and they care for you, but many friendships cannot withstand catastrophies of this proportion. So that's not the answer. The answer, I think, is what we're all trying to do here today, and that is gather together those of us who have similar problems so that we can support one another.

"We want to stretch out our hands to each other and say, 'Hey, it's okay. I know what it's like. We'll live through it.' We're going to help each other, and we're going to change the system, because we are the ones who make this country work."

I could feel that my listeners were receptive to the zeal in my voice. There are those who can stand on stage and be quietly objective. That was not my role. If I have a role and a gift in this world it is to present passion. I feel passionately and speak passionately, and in so doing I seem to be able to touch people.

Finally I said, "I hope to get this whole thing rolling to Washington, but I cannot do it alone. The San Francisco Mental Health Association cannot do it alone. The Task Force cannot do it alone, but we can surely do it together because the time has come and, by golly, we're going to make it work. Aren't we?"

"Yes! Yes!" shouted back the audience.

After our first public meeting, I conducted a medical ethics workshop, which was gratifying, but my primary objective at this stage was to reach the decision-makers in Washington to make them aware that there was a national tragedy caused by inadequate services in our society for brain-damaged victims.

When I was growing up my mother taught me, through her own example, that I owed it to myself and to society to help others. I now had the energy, the motivation, and the courage to pursue such altruism. I believed in my cause so much, and I believed in our political system so earnestly, that I had no hesitation in starting from the top. I began a letter-writing campaign to some of the highest officials in the land. Elatedly, I found I got a response from most of these men and women. This, in itself, is a persuasive acknowledgment of the average citizen's power in a democracy.

Senator Alan Cranston's reply was typical. He encouraged me to come to Washington, saying, "I hope to be able to meet with you and hear your story firsthand, my schedule permitting. In any event I would most definitely want you to meet with my legislative assistant for health, Louise Ringwalt."

I opened many doors into the Washington world myself, but I was also lucky to have friends who opened some special ones. For instance, Dr. Edward Clark, the chairman of the Department of Neurology at the hospital where I worked, told me that he knew Senator Hubert Humphrey and Vice President Walter Mondale personally. He gladly wrote to these men on my behalf and received replies from both Humphrey and Mondale stating they, or their aides, would be pleased to see me. (Several years later Dr. Clark, who had tried to help the brain-damaged, died of a brain tumor.)

My friend Nancy Lapham put me in touch with Caspar Weinberger, and he in turn wrote to Dr. Faye G. Abdellah, who was then the assistant surgeon general of the U.S. Public Health Service. In his letter to Dr. Abdellah, Weinberger wrote: "I would appreiate it very much if you could write to her [Anne Bashkiroff] with any suggestions you might have as to how the basic problem can be handled. . . . She is primarily interested in how she can help others in this dilemma. I hope this will not be too much trouble for you, but I really think this is an extremely good cause, and it certainly is one that has attracted a lot of attention here."

Dr. Abdellah referred me to other individuals and I found myself in a chain reaction, each person strengthening the chain with his support. My mail bolstered my optimism. If these busy and prominent people were taking the time to write to me, and even wanted to see me, then surely the problems of brain-damaged people could be surmounted.

We heard the President's Commission on Mental Health was going to be holding a hearing in San Francisco.

"Anne," said Barbara Cohen, "there might be a chance for you to testify before the Commission about the lack of services for brain-damaged people."

It was a slim chance. I sent in my application, knowing hundreds of individuals wanted to testify about numerous issues, and the Commission was only allowing two days of testimony for the entire western part of the United States. Less than fifty would be chosen to speak at the San Francisco public hearing.

I probably would never have had the chance to speak except for a series of synchronistic events that began to take place; it was almost as if I was destined to testify.

Douglas Watersteet, the national director of organization development for the National Mental Health Association, came to San Francisco from Washington to attend a conference. Libby Denebeim, the president of the San Francisco Mental Health Association, introduced him to me.

Doug was a moving train. He had been active in mental health issues for years and knew how to advance programs with a speed and style that was admirable. I told Doug I was prepared to go to Washington to lobby for our cause, and he promised to put me in touch with all the key people, including the First Lady, Rosalynn Carter, who was honorary chairperson of the President's Commission on Mental Health.

As we were talking about whom I should contact, Doug mentioned that a good friend of his, Dr. George Tarjan, professor of psychiatry at the University of California, Los Angeles, School of Medicine, had been selected to be on the President's Commission. (Later, Dr. Tarjan would serve as 1983 president of the American Psychiatric Association.)

"The name, George Tarjan, rings a bell," I said to Doug. "I can't imagine where I've heard it before."

"He's well known for his work with retarded children," explained Doug. "He's in charge of the UCLA Division of Mental Retardation and Child Psychiatry."

"His name sounds Armenian," I remarked.

"He's Hungarian, like my wife," said Doug, correcting me.

As soon as I heard "Hungarian" it clicked. "What a coincidence," I said. "Now I know why his name sounded so familiar. A Hungarian friend of mine who now lives in Caracas wrote about George Tarjan in his Christmas letter."

For a number of years Sasha and I received a Christmas holiday letter from Eric Haas, a man we had known in Shanghai, during the war. In his last letter Eric described a joyful reunion with a school classmate, George Tarjan. Tarjan, he wrote, was in Caracas to receive the highest civil decoration of Venezuela for his work with retarded children.

One man referred by two people, in two different parts of the world. It was too much of a coincidence to ignore. I promptly sent a letter to Dr. Tarjan, explaining how I knew both Eric Haas and Doug Waterstreet. I also told him how Doug was trying to arrange for me to meet Mrs. Carter and other distinguished people in the mental health field. I asked him, as boldly as I could, to assist me in my endeavors.

Dr. Tarjan's reply was compassionate and constructive. He wrote, "The full year's agenda of the President's Commission is not yet crystallized. It is for this reason that I am taking the liberty of bringing this matter to the attention of Dr. Thomas E. Bryant who is Chairperson of the Commission and chairs it whenever Mrs. Carter is absent. I know that he will give it his most thoughtful attention and I am confident that he will also speak about the situation to Mrs. Carter."

A letter soon arrived from Dr. Bryant on White House stationery asking me to send documentation of my experience with Sasha.

A few weeks later, while I was in Los Angeles visiting my sister, I arranged a meeting with Tarjan at his UCLA office. He listened attentively as I gave him more details of my experience with Sasha's illness. It was a valuable meeting. By now, the scheduled speakers for the San Francisco hearing of the President's Commission on Mental Health had already been chosen, but Tarjan must have felt that my story really needed to be heard because he exerted his influence as a commissioner to suggest to Dr. Bryant that I testify from the floor.

I then received another letter from Bryant, this one stating he hoped I would attend the San Francisco public hearing, although he cautioned that he couldn't guarantee there would be time for me to speak from the floor. I wasn't discouraged. It was an opportunity and I grabbed it.

The hearing was held in the Rose Room of the Sheraton Palace Hotel. Because of Rosalynn Carter's presence there were secret-service men everywhere. Before the session began I managed to introduce myself to Bryant, who kindly explained the procedure to me. "Everyone who wants to testify from the floor has to fill out a card," he said. "Fill out yours and send it in with the rest of the names. If I can I'll see that you get called." And he emphasized once again, "I can't promise your name will be chosen."

The large ballroom was packed to capacity. The commissioners were placed at a long table in the front of the room and cordoned off from the audience. Rosalynn Carter, with Bryant and Tarjan on either side of her, began the hearing by observing, "It's going to be a busy, very full day. I want you to know that we had over five hundred requests from people who wanted to testify. There's no way we could hear from five hundred people in one day, but we're really excited about the enthusiastic response."

By the end of the morning there were only three people chosen to testify from the floor. I was the third individual.

I had learned to overcome my tension in front of TV cameras and large groups, but there is something about speaking in front of the wife of the President of the United States that unsettles the nerve cord. When my name was announced I was a coiled spring, but halfway through my testimony I relaxed as I saw Bryant and Tarjan smiling at me, like mentors pleased with their protégée.

During the three minutes that I was allotted to give my speech I received three ovations. I was the only person at the hearing who spoke about Alzheimer's disease. Indeed, there were probably many people in the room who weren't even aware of the critical problems that face Alzheimer's patients and their families.

After my testimony there was a break. Immediately, George Tarjan got up, climbed over the rope barrier, and came across the room to congratulate me. Then he took my elbow and guided me toward Rosalyn Carter who greeted me warmly and thanked me for my testimony.

That afternoon I returned to work. As I sat at my typewriter my mind celebrated the knowledge I had made a significant contribution toward assisting Sasha and other brain-damaged victims.

My testimony was televised by Channel 2 *Action News* as part of a program they were presenting on the enormous cost of caring for brain-damaged patients. It was an excellent series but I strongly objected to the title they chose: "The High Cost of Insanity."

It was a matter of education. This title showed us, once again, that many people still didn't understand senile dementia is a physical organic brain disease, which happens to cause mental problems. It was an injustice to simplistically call these victims "insane."

Conversely, for years the professionals in the mental health field had been reluctant to pay any attention to brain-damaged victims because these patients had primarily physical disorders. Until the San Francisco Mental Health Association adopted my case, the specific emotional problems of brain-damaged patients had never been addressed either in California or anywhere in the country. The San Francisco MHA was the first mental health branch in the nation to accept the responsibility that although brain disorders were physical they also caused extreme mental conditions for the victims and their families, and therefore these individuals should also be included under their umbrella.

In August 1977, the Board of Directors of the Mental Health Association of San Francisco granted the Family Survival Task Force status as a Special Project, making our work one of the top priorities of the Association.

By now our group had also made several trips to Sacramento, the state capital, to lobby for comprehensive care for brain-damaged people in California. On one of our visits we met with Dr. Jerome Lackner, the director of the State Department of Health.

Dr. Lackner gave us good political advice: First, he said, we had to get the camel's nose under the tent. In political terms this meant a pilot program. Before even a pilot program could be established, he added, we should conduct a study to identify the needs of brain-damaged patients and their families. Then we could design a pilot program to meet those needs.

It was a political game. Our study had to prove to politicians beyond a reasonable doubt, said Dr. Lackner, that these families deserved aid before we could request legislation for a pilot program.

"You don't have to be a great scholar of social medicine to know damn well these families desperately need help," acknowledged Dr. Lackner, who had become a champion of our cause, "but first you have to prove a pilot program can work before you can extend the aid and push the camel the whole way."

To conduct a study we needed funding from the Department of Health. We knew such a request for funding would be more likely to pass if our group had the state-wide support of the California Mental Health Association. With the crucial cooperation of Peter DuBois, the executive director of the California Mental Health Association, we persuaded the CMHA to pass a resolution recognizing brain-damaged individuals as a distinct group. This recognition of our unique needs was a major accomplishment, and ultimately secured the funding for the study.

These achievements at the state level made me determined to also visit the politicians in Washington, but Sasha's expenses in the nursing home were consuming my savings and I couldn't afford to pay for such a trip. A dear woman friend, who wants to remain anonymous, offered to sponsor me.

It was arranged for me to travel to Washington with Peter DuBois of the CMHA, and Libby Denebeim, the president of the San Francisco MHA. I had never been to Washington, and the last time Libby saw the capital was twenty-five years earlier, shortly after her honeymoon. We arrived eager to see not only Washington's monuments, but also the inner offices of our government.

My spate of letter-writing had led to many appointments with congressmen or their aides, as well as important staffers of special committees. Peter and Libby had also set up appointments and altogether we had a hectic schedule. The three of us spoke to anyone who would listen to us.

We were a persuasive team. I had the ability to make people understand the issue because I could personalize the problems, and Peter and Libby were armed with cold facts to illustrate that what was happening to me was happening to people all over the country. In addition, they had the knowledge of laws and the political process.

Many who saw us were sympathetic and helpful, but we also found indifference. To some extent this indifference was understandable. Every month these politicians heard of new problems with various diseases until they developed "disease of the month" cynicism. Our job was to convince them our cause wasn't temporary, and couldn't be so easily dismissed.

I remember a meeting we had with a member of the Senate Finance Committee. The man we shook hands with was young, but he had risen rapidly on the political ladder. As we made our pitch he didn't hide his boredom. He implied he was fed up listening to these types of problems.

His hardened attitude angered me. "When did you last see your wife?" I asked him, noticing a wedding ring on his finger.

My question caught him off guard. "Why, this morning," he replied warily.

What I said next shocked him. It was meant to. Maybe he was fed up, but I was also fed up with people who thought brain damage was an esoteric issue that wouldn't touch their lives.

"Perhaps," I continued, "you should telephone your wife and see if she is all right. Brain damage is often caused by automobile accidents. Your wife might have been in a car accident today."

The young man's boredom stopped; he began paying attention to us. Then something happened that stressed my point further, in a more profound way than my harsh analogy. The man offered to telephone a colleague who, he said, might help us.

He was smiling as he made the telephone call, but what he heard on the other end of the line dramatically changed his expression. The smile dropped.

"I've just found out," he said, turning to us, "that my colleague is in the hospital. He had a stroke and has suffered brain damage."

Our trip to Washington was summed up in an article written by Tom Eastham, which appeared on the front page of the Los Angeles *Herald Examiner*. It was headlined: "The Bottom Line: Big Government Doesn't Always Turn Deaf Ear." In the piece Eastham quoted the following politicians.

Senator Edward Kennedy's health expert, Dr. Stewart Shapiro: "Mrs. Bashkiroff described her problem movingly. But while the story is personal, she showed the problem is broad and general—that of continuing care for people who have brain damage or are chronically ill. It impressed me, and it will impress my boss—Senator Kennedy."

Dr. Peter D. Fox, policy analyst for the Department of Health, Education, and Welfare: "We become so hardened to people coming in just wanting more money. This time we genuinely learned something. This problem has not been focused on and it obviously needs attention. I was simply not familiar with it."

Louise Ringwalt, health aide to Senator Alan Cranston: "When an individual comes to a congressional office it dramatizes and humanizes the kind of difficulties people have. We get a lot of letters, but we don't often see the people who are having such health troubles."

Vice President Walter Mondale's domestic advisor, James Dyke: "This kind of visit brings problems to our attention we haven't been aware of. Their visit caused us to contact other federal agencies to find out if there is indeed a problem and what might be done about it. We can safely say they brought the problem to the appropriate officials, and it will get appropriate concern."

Before we left Washington we also attended the annual meeting of the National Mental Health Association, where I once again met Rosalynn Carter. I had my photograph taken with her, and as I stood by her side I reflected upon how far I had traveled from my initial call to Jane Ophuls of the San Francisco MHA to tell her of my plight. That one call had been made from the bottom of a mountain. It had been an arduous climb but at last, I thought, maybe our goals were within reach.

On February 24, 1978, the Family Survival Project received the funds from the California Department of Health to conduct a study so we could assess the needs of irreversibly brain-damaged victims and their families.

On that day Sasha died.

Chapter 9

DESPAIR

Alexander Theodore Bashkiroff
A man who lived in history, who was history
A man who was soul and heart, a gentle man, a giver.
A man with a family that was his life
A man from another time, lost in the present;
        a memory for the past, timeless . . .
A man who has endured the hardships,
       the joys and the pain of life.
          A man at peace.

Nicky had told me he wanted to write a eulogy for his father, but on the day of Sasha's memorial service he hadn't prepared it.

"I'll do it right now," he said, as we stood in our kitchen.

"But we have to leave for the church soon," I protested. "There's no time."

"Don't worry, Mom," he assured me. "It won't take long."

Nicky completed the eulogy in less than five minutes. He knew exactly what he wanted to say.

Sasha died of heart failure, alone in a locked ward, miles away from us. I arranged for his body to be brought to a San

Francisco mortuary, and Nicky and I immediately went to the mortuary to see him. We found Sasha in a room by himself, lying as if in bed, with a sheet draped up to his chin. I could only see my husband's face, but the sight of it softened my sorrow. I no longer detected the fixed features of suffering; the craziness that had hung in his eyes and mouth had gone. I thought I even saw an amused look on his face as if he were telling me: See, I've thrown away the bad part.

I bent down, kissed him, and cradled his head, stroking his fine hair.

Then, I pulled back the sheet.

"Mom, what are you doing?" cried Nicky, alarmed I was disturbing the covering.

"Leave me alone. It's all right."

I took out one of Sasha's hands and held it in my own. When you love someone, there is usually a characteristic that identifies that person to you, and for me it was Sasha's hands. They were big hands, not handsome, but capable, and somehow commanding. I held onto Sasha's hand for a long time.

Within a few years this was the third death in my family. My father, my mother, and now my husband. When my parents died I mourned fully. The mourning settled like a cloud until I had emptied my grief and then it lifted. It wasn't as easy to mourn Sasha. I had lost him in bits and pieces as his brain left him, and my crying had been spread, as the disease spread, over months and years. Sasha had died many times, although his body had continued to live, and I had accepted long ago that I had become a widow, although society didn't recognize me as one. In this social limbo I had already completed my mourning, but because it was so extended I never felt I had decently mourned my husband at all.

How much can one grieve? How much can one cry? I don't know, but I confess by the time Sasha was officially pronounced dead I found it hard to relive all the tears I had already spent. But ah—we can be so righteous with mourning, and be made to feel so guilty if we don't comply with set standards. I remember after my mother died I was upset because her physician didn't act as if he cared.

This doctor took care of my mother while she was at the nursing home. At first she didn't like him because he talked to her as if she were a foolish child. My mother didn't put up with the doctor's condescending manner for long; her sickness never quelled her intelligence nor the speed of her retorts. She marched to the head nurse and said, "How dare he talk to me that way? Does he think I am stupid, senile? I have remembered more today than he will ever remember in his entire life!"

The head nurse had a talk with the doctor, and the doctor promptly delivered mother an apology. From then on a strong friendship developed between them, and my mother looked forward to his visits, saving stories to tell him.

I had also been in constant touch with this doctor during the last few months of my mother's life, and I had expected him to call and give me further details of how she died. When I didn't hear from him I wondered if he had feigned fondness for our family. I couldn't understand his abrupt silence, and in anger I called his office. I planned to scalp him, but before I could say anything he began, "Anne, I'm sorry. I know I should have telephoned you a long time ago but I have great difficulty dealing with death, and with Aida's death particularly. We became so close. She was like a mother to me. As I talk to you, I am crying . . ."

I ended up consoling him. I told him how important it was for me to hear that it was the *intensity* of his feelings that had prevented him from calling me, rather than the lack of them.

Now, after Sasha's death, I had a greater awareness of the complexity of mourning. To some people I must have seemed callous because I didn't appear to react to the death of my husband. But within my conscience I knew the epic journey of my bereavement.

Sasha had once told me he wanted to be cremated. He had

been ambivalent about a religious service, for he was not actively religious, attending church only once a year to commemorate his mother's death. Yet I couldn't part with him in a mortuary. His illness had affronted him at every level, and I felt it was vital that I now give him back his dignity.

My husband had been fond of one church, a small, exquisite Russian Orthodox cathedral, where we had Nicky christened. It was the oldest Russian Orthodox church in San Francisco, built in the 1860s. It was there I decided I could have a service of dignity and splendor.

We held our observance to Sasha on a March Sunday, after the normal worship service. I had no time to invite people formally, and merely called a few friends, and asked them to telephone others. To my surprise and pleasure, the church was crowded. Even George came.

Each guest was given a candle to hold, and the flames from these candles massed into a luminous galaxy. The smell of the burning candles mingled with the thick scent of incense, which the priest repeatedly tossed into the air from his brass and silver-plated censer as he moved about the cathedral. This ancient ritual of incense awakened all my senses, and the pureness of the cathedral's a cappella choir magnified these senses until the beauty of the service was etched into my heart forever.

The day was overcast, but once—while the choir was singing—the light swiftly changed and the stained-glass windows behind the altar scattered sunbeams into our faces. Heady with the power of prayer within the cathedral, Nicky and I saw this light and took it as a sign that Sasha's soul was acknowledged.

The priest spoke in Church Slavonic, except for Nicky's eulogy, which he read in English. The eulogy must have affected many men in the congregation, for afterwards they came up to me and said they hoped their children felt the same way about them as Nicky felt about his father.

Immediately following the service our guests were invited into the cathedral's hall for Russian food. As we ate we reminisced; mostly we spoke of Sasha's good times.

Two days later Sasha's ashes were dropped in the Pacific ocean, a private ceremony just for Nicky and me. We went down to the pier and boarded a small tugboat. The afternoon was clear with only a thin line of fog fingering the top of the Golden Gate Bridge. As we moved away from the shore, San Francisco's tall buildings divided the blue sky. Tourists on other boats took their pictures, and my memory returned to the time when I first saw San Francisco. The Golden Gate Bridge was my entrance to the United States from China, and as the ship passed under the bridge, I had tossed my Shanghai house key into the ocean below.

Sasha loved the sea. Nicky and I studied the white caps, trying to ignore the wreath that had been placed on the bench opposite us, but no matter what we talked about we were only too aware of this wreath, and the green bag of ashes inside its center. This was Nicky's father. This was my husband. This was all that was left.

Finally the tugboat stopped in a cove just past the Golden Gate Bridge, and the boat's owner asked, "Who wants to throw the wreath overboard?"

For a few seconds neither Nicky nor I responded. Then Nicky said, "I'll do it."

He took the wreath firmly in his hands and threw it, and as he did so the waiting seagulls swooped down. The boat pulled away. Nicky and I immediately held each other, mother and son clinging, crying.

As the boat returned toward the San Francisco piers, we stood by the rail and watched the wreath bobbing in the ocean, the seagulls still encircling it. My thoughts chased the waves: What is this? Is this all there is to eternity? Tears, ashes, and seagulls fighting for remains?

So much sifts through the mind at a time like this—critical as well as caring thoughts—but ultimately all these thoughts were overpowered by the sea's omnipotent spirituality. One red carnation in the wreath caught the sunlight and my imagination. In this floating flower I saw only grace. I kept my eyes on it, a fragile ruby that became smaller and smaller until it faded into a dewdrop. Then it disappeared.

Toward the end of Sasha's illness I was told my husband's symptoms were indicative of Alzheimer's disease, but at that time there was little educational material available on Alzheimer's, and I knew nothing about the possibility that the disease might be hereditary.

A definitive diagnosis of Alzheimer's rests on finding abnormal structures in the brain tissues, and this is usually only confirmed in death through an autopsy. When Sasha died, the doctor didn't suggest an autopsy, and although I would have been reluctant to have ordered this last violation of Sasha's body, I know now that for my family's sake it would have been better to have had an autopsy and positively identified Sasha's sickness. If future research reveals a hereditary factor is involved in Alzheimer's, then Nicky, and any children he might have, will always wonder whether or not Sasha really had this disease.

Sasha's cause of death was listed as heart failure. When a nursing home patient dies, most doctors cite the immediate cause of death—such as pneumonia or heart failure—although the real basis of death may be something else entirely—such as organic brain disease, or an accidental injury. This means the U.S. Vital Statistics tables are misleading because they don't accurately reflect the large number of deaths due to these primary causes.

Dr. Robert N. Butler, head of the geriatrics department at Mount Sinai School of Medicine, New York, and Pulitzer prize-winning author of *Why Survive? Being Old in America*, estimates that dementias are the fourth leading cause of death in the United States.

In a report in the journal *Aging*, Butler urged, "We need to reform death certificates to reflect the primary cause of death so that epidemiological studies will be based on accurate data. As research progresses in the area of Alzheimer's disease/senile dementia, epidemiology will take on even greater importance. We must ensure that the raw data from which epidemiologists work is valid and reliable."

Sasha was dead, but my crusade wasn't. I was now chairman of the Family Survival Project, the project that had been given special status by the San Francisco Mental Health Association, and we were more determined than ever to establish a program that would benefit all brain-damaged victims and their families.

Until our Washington trip, we had considered seeking congressional action for brain-damaged adults, particularly since Marjorie Guthrie, the widow of the famous folksinger and composer Woody Guthrie, had already stirred the congressional conscience about Huntington's disease.

Marjorie had become my friend, as well as my inspiration. We had instant rapport, for both of us had travelled through tragedy. In 1967 Woody Guthrie died of Huntington's, a hereditary brain disorder, but for years he was misdiagnosed as an alcoholic or schizophrenic, and was in and out of mental hospitals before the true diagnosis of Huntington's disease was made.

Since his death, Marjorie had worked continuously to make life easier for other victims. It was because of her efforts that the Commission for the Control of Huntington's Disease and Its Consequences was mandated by Congress to study the medical and social problems of the disease.

This commission was a pioneering step for victims of Huntington's, and we had hoped to follow Marjorie's footsteps and amplify her success, but while we were in Washington, we were warned it would be a difficult and lengthy process to get action on a national level for all brain-damaged people.

Congressman Phillip Burton, whom I had met through Clara Shirpser Levy, the former Democratic national committee-woman for California, advised: "Congressional action takes time. If you want a more immediate answer to your problems, then I tell you what you should do. Take your energy and focus it at the state level. Get state legislation passed in California and start a pilot program."

We took his advice. Although we had already begun work on introducing state legislation, we had not focused totally on this goal. The members of our Family Survival Project had also spent time researching loopholes in laws, had made attempts to change insurance policies, had chased private funding as well as public funding, and all in all had dispersed energy and resources in a hundred and one directions.

I had even contacted an eminent lawyer, Frederick Furth, to see if I could, as a private citizen, sue the City of San Francisco and the State of California for unequal protection, showing that social welfare legislation didn't protect middle-income families.

Furth devoted time to my case, but decided I didn't have a practical legal recourse. He also concluded: Win new legislation at the state level.

The turning point toward winning such legislation came when we were given the grant from the California State Department of Health to study the effects of brain damage on families. We knew this study could directly lead to legislative action because it enabled the state to evaluate the fiscal aspects of the problem.

We hired a private research firm, Steve Thompson and Associates, to conduct the study. I had met Steve Thompson at Mayor George Moscone's office, and had persuaded him to attend a Family Survival meeting. From then on he became one of our staunchest advocates.

At last we had the chance to win one major victory. We wanted to make California the model state with the first piece of legislation in the country designed to help victims of all forms of organic brain damage.

As the Thompson study got underway, my personal life took a roller-coaster course; unfortunately, after Sasha's death I was more down than up.

One of my happier moments was when I won an award. The San Francisco *Examiner* participated in the American Institute of Public Service's Jefferson Award Program for community service, and each year they named six local citizens who had served to benefit the San Francisco community. I was honored to be one of those citizens. In March 1978, only a few weeks after Sasha died, I was presented with the Jefferson Award for my work with brain-damaged victims and their families.

Up until then I hadn't really thought of myself as a citizen activist. However, around the same time I attended a party for Jane Fonda to celebrate her movie "Coming Home," which had just premiered. It was a small gathering, held at the home of Lacey Fosburgh, a writer, and David Harris, writer and political activist. Most of the guests were involved in social change, and introductions were inclined to include not only one's name, but also one's cause.

In this milieu, a woman came up to me and said, "Are you an activist too?" I thought: What's she talking about? Then I realized: I guess I am. So I said, "Yes," and was surprised to hear the assertiveness in my voice.

At one point during the party I noticed that Jane Fonda kept glancing in my direction. People are always telling me I look like somebody they know and I thought perhaps Jane had mistaken me for someone else. I went up to her and said, "Jane, why are you staring at me?"

"Because," she replied, "you have such beautiful eyes."

She said it with such sincerity I was flattered. "Jane, coming from you that's a real compliment!"

I left the party feeling as if I had been given a tonic.

Keeping busy was one way of keeping my mind away from my problems. I was happiest when I was caught up in some sort of social whirl. But there were weekends when no friends were available, and when even the telephone didn't ring. And there were many months when life seemed to consist of work and nothing else.

One of Sasha's favorite sayings was, "Nature abhors a vacuum." He was an optimistic person who believed that when life becomes empty and sad, there is always something good "just around the corner" to fill the void.

This concept gave me hope. Until Sasha's head became a vacuum. Until his death, when the part of my life that had been married to him became a vacuum . . . and nothing entered my life to replace this emotional loss. As time went by I began to wonder: Isn't there anything good ahead of me? Am I to live out my life alone?

In a *Journal of Clinical Psychiatry* article about brain-damaged patients, Dr. Muriel D. Lezak wrote: "Most family members who live with a characterologically altered brain injured patient suffer depression. For some, depression occurs as a chronic pall on their lives that continues even after the patient's death—not as mourning, but as a permanently fixed emotional burden."

I suspect for a long time I carried that burden. I wasn't always aware of the weight, and often I'd regain my natural optimism. Friends would exclaim, "Your mood is so exuberant." At these times I expected things to go well, but when the days and months passed and my expectations were not met, then the burden returned.

The more alone I felt, the more my life revolved around George's visits. It wasn't a one-sided relationship; I think in many ways we upheld each other because George was the type of man who liked to be "mothered," and he enjoyed the attention I lavished upon him.

"If only we had met earlier," he would say. "I've never known anyone like you. You're unique." Then he would shrug and add, "Everything in life is timing."

I knew George was not ready to remarry, and I wasn't sure I wanted to marry George or anyone else either. All I wanted was to love him and be loved in return. But lamentably I became increasingly dependent upon that love. It became my only sustenance. When I was waiting for him to call I'd think: My well-being is measured by the sound of his voice. How can I give him this awesome responsibility? I'd scold myself again and again: I shouldn't give him this power over me.

No amount of self-scolding lessened my dependency upon this man. George had come into my life when Sasha left it, and by these circumstances alone I felt that Sasha, George, and I were forever linked. I had been in love with Sasha. I was enamored with George. He became my mythical support, the last vestige of somebody who cared for me. One day I wrote, "Sasha is dead, dead, dead. That's it! I will have to deal somehow with Sasha's death if I let go of George."

Oh God, I didn't want to be so alone. Nature should arrange it so nobody is so alone. In my blackest minutes I'd accept: I don't belong to anybody. There is no one to tell me yes or no. I'm not under anybody's control.

Maybe some women envy or strive for such freedom but for me—a widow—this freedom was too raw. I needed limitations, somebody to care enough about me to say, "Don't do this because it's not good for you."

"La solitude est plus facile quand on est deux." I read this and thought how true; it was easy for me to have solitude when I was part of a couple, but as single person solitude was becoming more and more difficult.

I watched the clock pass many a three A.M. Several nights when I couldn't sleep I thought about my mother. Although we didn't always get along my mother knew me as nobody else did. I missed her. When we're young we think we don't need answers from mothers. Now I reflected: If she were here I would listen to her—things I didn't hear before, or wouldn't allow myself to hear.

My bed became my mother's womb. I didn't want to leave it. In these moments of depression I was outside the mainstream of life; the lives of other people continued, but mine rested in a bed, suspended.

I sensed my separateness from the world in the sound of the bedside clock as I purposely put myself in a dead center of nothingness. I was all alone . . . tick, tick, tick. Too often the ticking in my head became louder and louder, and my body became heavier and heavier. I felt as if I couldn't move. It would take all my mental and physical strength to break away from this self-hypnotic state. Usually when I became physically active the depression would automatically lift, but there were times when it would remain a clinging gauze over my brain for the rest of the day.

I regarded these depressions as disturbing but temporary interruptions to my life. For months after Sasha's death I coped as I had always done. I continued to work hard, both at my hospital job and for the Family Survival Project.

My job at Children's Hospital was one of my anchors. After working there twenty years I had been given certain powers, and a prestige position. I felt happy and secure in this niche. Then suddenly the hospital had a face-lift. There was a change in administration and a change in my responsibilities. My new work at the hospital demanded a knowledge of financial affairs, an area I knew little about. Day after day I came home depleted.

At the same time my relationship with Nicky had become pulverized. Ever since his return to California we had been at odds with one another. Sasha's illness had disrupted Nicky's life to such an extent he had lost interest in becoming an architect, and quit U.C. Berkeley after only one quarter. For

over a month he stayed home, moody, restless, not really
knowing what to do with his life. Eventually he found work as
a carpenter and then obtained a contractor's license.

His personal life was also as addled as my own. In the same
way that I tried to use George as my source of solace, Nicky also
tried to escape from his problems through women. Shortly after
Sasha died, Nicky got engaged to a woman he had only known
for a few weeks.

Initially, I thought marriage would be good for him. I
believed this was his chance to be happy. I also hoped that a
father-in-law would give Nicky a feeling of having a father-
figure in his life again.

Shortly before the wedding date I got a call from Nicky telling
me he had met another woman and was in love with her.

"I've made a mistake, Mom," he said. "I want to break my
engagement. Can you help me?"

In hindsight I probably should have helped him but I didn't
have anything left in me to aid anybody, so I said, "You must
deal with this yourself. You're old enough to get engaged. You
should be old enough to get disengaged without my interfer-
ence."

Nicky got married a month later. On his wedding day he
looked like a sacrificial lamb being led to the altar. He knew he
was making a mistake, and I probably knew it too, and yet all I
told him was, "Many people get nervous on their wedding day.
Things will work out."

They didn't work out. The marriage didn't last and during
the time they were married Nicky became morose and withdrawn. I rarely saw him. We got to the point where we couldn't
talk to each other, even on the telephone, without fighting.

We fought mostly over why he wasn't visiting me, or being
kind to me, or helping me in any way. What I didn't understand
was that just as I had become an empty vessel because of
Sasha's illness and death, so had Nicky. We both had become so
weak there was no way we could support each other.

As the arguments increased with Nicky, and my job became too difficult, I clung to the only other anchor I knew: George. Then that mainstay was also pulled away.

On a Saturday morning, the telephone rang. "You don't know me," said a woman, "but George is a friend of mine. He told me about you, and I would like to meet you. Can you see me for lunch today?"

She suggested a restaurant, and since I didn't have any plans I accepted her invitation. It was only after I hung up that I had an uneasy feeling. Although I had met a few of George's friends, I wondered why one of them would want to see me privately. I couldn't contact George and ask him about her because he was out of town for the weekend.

I arrived at the restaurant early. The place was small, pleasant, but nearly empty. I chose a seat at a corner table near the window and informed the waitress I was expecting company. Five minutes later I saw a tall, angular-framed woman enter, wearing a blue knitted suit that was tight at the hips. She stopped to talk to the waitress, and then looked in my direction. As she came towards me her hips undulated.

"You must be Anne Bashkiroff," she said, standing over me. She was probably younger than I, but her complexion was coarse, and the eye make-up too vivid for daytime.

She sat down, shook out the napkin, and got straight to the point of why she wanted to meet me; she didn't waste time in niceties. "Are you and George lovers?"

Her voice pierced my body and chilled it. My only defense was to reply haughtily, "Why are you asking me this?"

"Because I am having an intimate relationship with him, and if you were too, I would have every reason to be jealous of you." She actually smiled at me as she said this.

I don't know why I didn't get up and leave, but instead I gripped the menu as if it were my salvation.

She went on to tell me she met George two months ago, that

they immediately felt passion for each other, and it hadn't been difficult to entice him into bed.

"The poor man was so starved for affection," she said, her eyes watching me for any reaction. "He's been alone for so long. I am sure he told you about his wife's tragic death."

I didn't respond. My face and heart were stiff. She continued her monologue, the cruelty of her intent now only too obvious.

In explicit details she described their sex life, what he did to her, what she did to him. She left little to the imagination, taunting me with vulgarities. She didn't even bother to pause as the waitress served us.

From her purse she then pulled out a calendar, and flicked it to the month of December. Heavy red crosses marked most of the days.

"Let me see," she said, thrusting the calendar in front of me. "George came to my house Monday, Tuesday, Thursday . . ."

The crosses blurred. I thought: How did he fit me in?

She was pitiless. I don't know why George mentioned my name to her, but she no longer pretended to have any other reason for seeing me than to abort my dreams. George, she said, loved only her. She believed they would soon get married.

I walked away from the restaurant flattened. It was like experiencing another death. At that moment I felt I had not only lost George, but I had also lost my respect for him, and for myself.

As soon as I got home I called the psychologist who had been treating me and told her what had just happened. She was appalled and concerned, and kept telephoning me throughout the weekend to try and calm me down.

On Monday morning, at eleven o'clock, George called my office. "Hello, how are you?" he said, in his usual light-hearted tone.

"I need to see you," I replied curtly.

"I don't know if I can make it tonight."

"I don't know if you can," I said, mocking him, "but you will. It's for your own good."

I knew I had him worried. George hated confrontations; his favorite cliché was "don't rock the boat."

"You had better come," I repeated.

"You are certainly putting it in succinct terms," he noted, annoyed. "All right, I'll be over at six o'clock."

George greeted me with a kiss on the cheek. I led him into the living room, and waited until he was settled in a chair before I asked, "Did you have a nice weekend?"

"Yes thank you, very nice."

"Do you have anything special to tell me?"

"No . . ."

"Are you sure?"

Looking directly at me he said, "I'm sure."

"In that case," I responded, my chest heaving with emotion, "I have something to tell you."

I didn't spare him, any more than I had been spared. I described the woman, the pet names she told me he called her, and some of their choicest sexual encounters.

George finally stopped me. He jumped up from the sofa, agitated. "Look," he said, his hands flailing the air, "I'm sorry you had to be involved in this. I'll put an end to the relationship with the woman right now."

He rushed toward the hallway. I ran after him. "Stay and talk to me," I pleaded. "Don't leave me like this."

"I can't stay. I have to go."

I wanted some explanation, no matter what it was, some assurance he still cared for me, no matter how little it was. He left.

The next day George returned and this time we talked. He said he had looked in the mirror and hated what he saw. What he had done, he admitted, was despicable.

For the next two weeks my relationship with George returned

to normal—except I didn't heal. I decided my psychologist wasn't helping me and told her, "I'm fine. I don't need you any more."

"Please," she argued, "I feel you could still benefit from these sessions." But I withdrew from her, without being fair to either of us, and went instead to see a psychiatrist who had been recommended to me. I didn't give this man time to understand my fragile frame of mind.

One evening after George left my home I thought, to hell with it! Everything that had given me peace of mind or hope in life seemed to have been obliterated. I reasoned: Why keep suffering about George, about Nicky, about the work I hadn't completed that day in the office? Who needs this? I don't need this. I'm not accountable to anybody. It's just me alone in this world . . . Why should I keep going?

My internist usually gave me only a month's supply of tranquilizers and sleeping pills, but on my last visit he had given me a three-month supply. I stayed awake all night, my mind toying with fat pills in fat containers.

It was a cold decision. I wasn't hysterical, just abysmally tired. I'm sure I didn't really want to die, but it was the only way I knew to terminate all problems.

In the morning I went to the bathroom, tipped the pills into my hand, and methodically started swallowing. Some pills fell on the floor and I picked them up and swallowed those too.

I climbed back into bed and called my sister in Boulder Creek, California. I told Betty I was feeling sad and asked her not to contact George, but to take care of Nicky.

I must have tried to call somebody else—I don't remember who. I fell asleep with the telephone off the hook, near my hand.

My sister, in the meantime, realized something was wrong and called my friend Mary. When Mary dialed my number she kept getting a busy signal. Mary had consoled me through many a crisis, and it didn't occur to her that this time the crisis might be more urgent than the others. After a few minutes she stopped trying to reach me, thinking she would talk to me later in the day.

When I didn't turn up for work, my colleagues also telephoned and they, too, turned to other matters after hearing the busy signal. It would have ended there except for a fluke.

Nicky was now a general contractor who worked out in the field, so it was usually impossible to reach him during the day, and he hardly ever called me. On this day though he telephoned my office in the morning. When he found out I hadn't gone to work, and hadn't given any reason for my absence, Nicky headed for my home. He found me unconscious.

Nicky immediately called an ambulance and I was raced to the hospital. Shortly after I arrived, I suffered cardiac arrest. Later I was told my chances for survival had been fifty-fifty. I was also made to face another fact: Such an overdose could have left me permanently brain-damaged, an ironic possibility I hadn't considered.

Chapter 10

THE SPIRIT OF SURVIVAL

When I became conscious I saw my son's face bending over me. Nicky kissed me gently and after a moment or two asked, "Do you want to see George? He's been at the hospital off and on since you were admitted, and he's outside waiting now."

I remember saying, "I'll see him if he wants to see me."

George entered, held my hand, and said, "I love you. I always will."

A suicide attempt stirs up the mud of guilt; people searched for something or someone to blame. Many friends said, "After Sasha's death, Anne had no one to live for." Nicky said, "I'm not going to take this guilt. It's not my fault." George said, "That was a very hostile act."

I spent my time reassuring everyone that nobody was responsible. I was the one who played with pills, who opened my mouth and carefully swallowed each one.

I also repeatedly heard, "How could you? You were so strong. How could you? You were the one who gave us our strength. How could you? You're the Rock of Gibraltar."

At first I sloughed off these comments and jokingly told people, "Well, it's all part of my research for the Family Survival Project."

The joke was on me. Good strong me. The person who nobody thought would attempt such a silly thing. However, after a while the punch line evaded me. I could not bear to hear one more person tell me how strong I was supposed to be.

Then I heard something that allowed me to reevaluate the double-edged sword of weakness and strength. While I was at the hospital I called Dr. George Tarjan, the psychiatrist who had helped me testify before Rosalynn Carter. I needed some medical advice, which he gave me, and as we were talking I mentioned I was troubled by my friends' concept that I was immune to despair.

"Anne," said my valued adviser, "we're all at risk."

His statement, to me, was profound.

My suicide attempt not only brought out the guilt in me and others, but it also evoked other complex feelings. One night we had a dinner party on my hospital bed with Nicky and some of my friends. We drank champagne and my friends got giddy with the euphoria that overcomes people when they discover someone is living, when he or she could have been dead. There was an aura of New Year's Eve in my room, except the celebrating went beyond that; my friends acted as if they were bringing in another life.

"Anne, what are you going to do now?" said one man.

"Yes Anne," said another. "You've got this second chance. You should do something fantastic."

Their message was: Okay kid, you've survived this experience. You could have been dead. You could have lost everything. Now you've got this whole new life ahead of you. Aren't you *lucky*? Prove how lucky you are. Do something *extraordinary*.

I was still in never-never land, not quite ready to enter the world, let alone conquer it, but I drank more champagne and joined their game. "I'm going around the world," I said.

I said the most idiotic things. I was going to sell my house, spend all my money. There wasn't anything I wasn't going to do.

I saw my son observing me. His face was unsmiling, far removed from our carnival. The next morning as Nicky walked me up and down the hospital corridor for my daily exercise he said, "Mother, I don't like the way you're reacting to all this. You're up in the clouds, not dealing with reality."

It took my son, who had been through his own nightmare because of my suicide attempt, to sensitize me. We stopped walking and he took both my hands in his. "You're not making plans to change your life to see this never happens again," he stressed solemnly. "I'm very concerned about it. I think you should go away to some sanitarium and rest and think."

He returned me to my bed and I lay very still and decided he was right. I knew I was depleted, that the years of caring for Sasha had finally caught up with me, and I required somebody, at least for a short time, to look after me.

Later that day I told my psychiatrist about Nicky's suggestion and he thought it was an excellent idea. It was arranged for me to attend a six-week therapy program at the Menninger Clinic in Topeka, Kansas. My psychiatrist recommended Menninger not only because it was considered one of the best health treatment centers in the country, but also because he believed it would be better for me to be amongst strangers, far removed from the San Francisco mental health community where I was too well known.

So I went to Topeka. I stayed at a cottage on the Menninger grounds with sixteen other patients and discovered each one of them had also attempted suicide. That's the shocker. You think you're special, that your attempt at suicide is special, and then you find out everyone in the room has done the same thing.

At first it was hard for me to adjust to the clinical routine and to live so familiarly with people I had never met before. All the patients were encouraged not to have any secrets from one another; we were there to learn from each other, and yet a couple of weeks had to pass before I accepted the idea that an eighteen-year-old had as much to add to my life experience as I did to hers.

For a while I thought I had made a mistake in coming to the clinic. I wanted to return to California and be with my friends. Then one morning fall turned into winter. I woke up to find that Topeka had been stilled by snow.

There were huge, magnificent trees on the Menninger grounds. Fall had stripped them of their leaves but now their massive limbs reached up to the sky embracing the snow that had fallen from it. Soft sunlight slanted over this white world, highlighting the brilliant red cardinals that swooped between the trees. The only other sign of life came from the chicadees, their gray bodies and dark black heads standing out like punctuation marks in this snowy landscape.

As soon as I could I went for a walk in the snow. My feet crunched into the powder. Looking around me I felt that everything—including myself—had been caught by surprise. Nature had given us no option but to view life from a new perspective. Nature had also demanded that life pause temporarily; the trees were obliged to stay covered with snow until it was right for them to awaken again with spring. There was a message in this. To me it was: Stop. Just as the trees are using this time to rest, rest your soul too.

That night I couldn't help but think how strange it was that my family had come from Siberia where snow was so much a part of their lives, and here I was in Topeka, Kansas, the navel of America, feeling suddenly at peace as if the snow had somehow healed me.

I pray to God I'll never attempt suicide again. I pray nothing will ever seem that hopeless again, but even if I should find myself on another ill-fated path, I now know enough to ask for help. And I pray we'll all remember to maintain a grasp on those who could slip . . .

After I left Topeka I heard that two of the patients in the Menninger program did try again. This time they died.

We are all at risk.

I never went back to my job after I returned to California, but I did continue to participate in the Family Survival Project. In my absence Jane Ophuls had taken over as chairman, and I was given the position of honorary chairman.

My cloistered weeks at the Menninger Clinic didn't instantly erase all problems, but they did ease them. It took time for me to improve my relationship with Nicky, just as it took time for me to put my relationship with George into perspective, and accept new male friends.

My love for Nicky had never diminished; he had always been the most vital part of my life, the part of me that had given life, not just existed in it, and it had hurt beyond expression when Nicky and I were pulled apart by our family tragedy. Both my son and I had to have more therapy before we eventually broke down the hostilities between us and became close again.

Immediately after my suicide attempt I found some people avoided me, or acted self-conscious in front of me. I think they actually feared me because they feared what I had done: I had dabbled in death. I had become vulnerable and people didn't want to get near me in case they exposed their own vulnerability.

If anything, my suicide attempt made me more acutely attuned to the emotional penalties families face when a noncurable disease pushes every member of that family into a seemingly never-ending tunnel marked No Exit.

When Steve Thompson's study on brain-damaged victims was published it confirmed that the personal anguish I had suffered with Sasha was not an isolated case. In response to a questionnaire Thompson sent families, one person wrote, "There were just the two of us. After ten years of full responsibility, when I was seventy, I began to 'fall apart.' No one cared. I had no social life. Old friends avoided me . . . and I drank too much . . . heavy depression and suicide attempts."

Thompson's study for the Family Survival Project also revealed that it wasn't uncommon for brain-damaged victims to be thrown out of nursing homes. It wasn't uncommon for families to become financially destitute because they couldn't pay for the care. And it wasn't uncommon for people to have trouble obtaining an accurate diagnosis of the patient's condition. A number of patients, reported Thompson, were actually misdiagnosed and labeled psychotic or schizophrenic because they showed "odd" behavior, when in fact the odd behavior was a direct symptom of neurological brain damage.

The Thompson study concluded that far too often not only the brains of the victims were destroyed, but also the lives of the people who cared for these patients.

In addition, the study made a strong political statement. Public policy, it said, discriminates against brain-damaged adults. "The only explanation for this social and financial inequity," the study added, "is that crippled, retarded and mentally ill people have secured public supported services after years of forceful, organized political action on their behalf. Brain-damaged adults have—until recently—had no such advocacy."

Well we now had the advocacy. The Thompson study proved there was a problem. The political clout of the Family Survival Project was recognized, and the pressure of my voice and all the other voices that were asking society to respond to the needs of brain-damaged victims and their families finally achieved the result we had dearly wanted.

On September 27, 1979, Governor Jerry Brown signed California Assembly Bill 1043, authored by Assemblyman Art Agnos, which established a pilot program for brain-damaged

victims and their families, to be administered by the Family
Survival Project.

The bill was co-sponsored by Assemblymen Willie Brown,
Gerald Felando, Leroy Greene, Louis Papan, and Maxine
Waters, and Senators Barry Keene and Milton Marks.

It was landmark legislation, not only because it was the first
piece of legislation in the country to fund a program for the
families of victims of all forms of organic brain disorders, but
also because it officially acknowledged the specific economic
and social problems of brain-damaged people.

With this funding, the Family Survival Project was able to
implement a pilot program in San Francisco and the surrounding counties that provided family support groups as well as
financial, legal, medical, and personal advice, plus much-
needed low-cost respite care in the home. Vital information
was consolidated into a centralized source so that a family only
had to make one telephone call, rather than the hundreds of
calls I underwent attempting to find help for Sasha.

During the last few years, our program has saved families
time, frustration, unnecessary foreclosures on homes, unnecessary divorces, and other inappropriate steps, and most of all it
has lessened their heartache and offered hope. Our services
have been offered through a voucher system, and families
contribute to the cost based on their ability to pay.

The program was everything I had wanted for others,
everything my hard-earned knowledge had told me was needed
if families were to survive with the dignity that both Sasha and
I were denied. When Sasha became ill I couldn't find anyone
who could advise me about the ramifications of caring for a
brain-damaged husband, and without this guidance I made
mistakes.

I have many disturbing memories: The lies I felt I had to tell
Sasha. The anger and fear I could not always contain. My

arguments with my son. Allowing Sasha to drive a car. Blunders and misjudgments. There was so much I didn't know.

Yet although I live with regrets, I also now live with the recognition that my agonized journey was not in vain. I once told a newspaper reporter, "As I fought my battle alone, I promised that all this suffering and sacrifice would not go to waste. I would use my expertise to help others."

In September 1980, the Family Survival Project cut its cord from the Mental Health Assocation and was incorporated as a non-profit organization. I became one of its board members. Today when I attend a board meeting of our Family Survival Project I often think back to that first meeting before the Mental Health Assocation's Community Assessment Committee, when I related my experience with Sasha and demanded something be done for all brain-damaged people. Today, there are family support groups. Today, a family can find counseling and emotional shelter. Today, no one has to struggle in isolation any more, and for that, and for all the progress we have made, I am thankful.

My character has withstood a storm and has been polished by it. I think I am a better person than I started out to be. It can take time spent in dark hours before we can see clearly. When I married Sasha I was judgmental, impatient, and held flimsy interpretations of life. In order to assert myself or prove a point, I could sometimes be insensitive, tossing out comments that hurt others; my actions didn't always contribute to the happiness of friends and acquaintances.

Now, having gone through so much trauma with Sasha, compassion has become an integral part of my character. I cannot listen to the problems of others without the reaction of "What can I do?" Very few of us go through life without some sort of crisis touching us. No one knows what's ahead from one minute to the next, and I believe none of us can afford to turn away from a stranger's problems, because tomorrow we may need the very help we have denied that stranger.

I also believe giving has a boomerang effect; whatever we send out comes back to us.

If there is to be any meaning to my life—and to Sasha's life—and if there is to be any meaning to the inherent promise Sasha and I treasured as immigrants entering America, then it has to lie in the ultimate art of caring for one another.

Sasha had one other story he used to tell me about his boyhood years. Near their estate in Samara there was a home for mentally disturbed people, or as the Russians describe them, *dushevno bolnie*, the soul-sick. When spring came these men and women used to take a daily walk across a lengthy meadow of new green grass, walking one in front of the other as if in a parade.

From a knoll near their home, Sasha and his brothers could look down on the meadow and often the boys would stop their playing and watch this march of the soul-sick. The brothers had intense curiosity about these people because they had been told they were "different."

Once, on a dare, the boys followed the walkers, staying a safe distance of several yards behind them until a woman with gray hair, who had been singing softly as she walked, turned and saw them. She immediately smiled and beckoned the brothers to come close.

As they approached she looked at the smallest boy and asked, "What is your name, little one?"

"Sasha," he replied shyly. Then, feeling brave because his two older brothers were by his side, Sasha said, "And what is your name?"

The woman bent down and picked one of the blue flowers growing wild in the meadow. She offered the flower to Sasha. "Nezabudka." ("Forget-me-not.")

Years later, when Sasha became brain-damaged, I used to have to gain admittance to the last home where he was placed through a locked iron gate. Intertwined in that gate was a trail of blue flowers.

I mie tebya, Sashinka, nekogda ne zabudim.

And we shall never forget you, dear Sasha.

ANNE BASHKIROFF:
AWARDS AND MILESTONES

1977. Represented the Family Survival Task Force and testi-
fied before First Lady Rosalyn Carter. She founded the Family
Caregiver's Alliance with the help of San Francisco Mayor Art
Agnos.

1978. The National Jefferson Award from the Institute of Public
Service.

1987. Certificate of Recognition from the Senate of the State of
California.

1987. Certificate of Honor from the B'nai B'rith's Anti-Defama-
tion League's "Woman on the Move" award.

1988. Jane S. Ophuls Award in appreciation of her leadership,
inspiration and support as Founder & Honorary Chair of Family Survival Project San Francisco.

1993. Top Bay Area Volunteers Award by Points of Light Cel-
ebration.

1994. Benny Award from the Women's International Center.

1995. Finalist, Rosalynn Carter Institute Caregiving Award.

1996. KGO-TV (ABC) Salute to Anne Bashkiroff.

1997. Cable 34: "Everybody's Angel" interviewed by Pari Livermore.

1998. Founder's Award, Alzheimer's Association, Chicago, Ill.

1999. Nominated for the Presidential Medal of Freedom, the highest civilian award in the nation by Thomas Eastham, VP, William Randolph Hearst Foundation.

1999. Rosalynn Carter Institute Caregiving Award, Georgia Southwestern State University.

2000. William R. Pothier Award, "Lives of Accomplishment," SF Senior Center.

2002. Certificate of Special Congressional Recognition "in recognition of outstanding and invaluable service to the community."

2005. Genesis Award, given to the pioneers who helped shape the Alzheimer's Association at their 25th Anniversary. Yasmin Khan, Rita Hayworth's daugher with Prince Ali Khan, presented the award.

ABOUT FAMILY
CAREGIVER ALLIANCE

History

Nearly 30 years ago, a small task force of families and community leaders in San Francisco (including Anne Bashkiroff and Suzanne Harris) came together to create support services for those struggling to provide long-term care for a loved one who did not "fit" into traditional health systems: adults with Alzheimer's disease, stroke, Parkinson's, traumatic brain injuries, and other debilitating disorders. The diagnoses were different, but the families shared common challenges: isolation, lack of information, few community resources, and drastic changes in family roles.

The task force's early efforts had three lasting results: the formation of Family Caregiver Alliance (FCA, formerly known as the Family Survival Project); the genesis of a statewide network of Caregiver Resource Centers; and the beginnings of a national movement to recognize the immense contribution of family caregivers to the long-term health care of the ill and elderly in our country.

National, State, and Local Programs

For residents of the six-county San Francisco Bay Area, FCA provides caregivers with information, publications, educational programs, care planning, legal consultations, individual and group

181

counseling, and assistance with respite care. FCA's popular Caregiver Retreats and Camps for Caring are examples of innovative programs that help caregiving families. FCA has received national and international recognition for "Best Practices" in caregiver support.

FCA is also the lead agency for California's statewide system of Caregiver Resource Centers, each modeled on the FCA program. In that role, FCA assists the California Department of Mental Health in documenting needs and services for caregivers throughout California.

In 2001, FCA established the National Center on Caregiving to advance the development of high-quality, cost-effective programs and policies for caregivers in every state in the country. Through the NCC, the Alliance publishes a wide variety of studies and reports and assists caregivers in locating support services throughout the nation.

FCA programs are funded by foundation grants, the state of California, the Administration on Aging, program participants, and donations.

CAREGIVING: STRATEGIES FOR DEALING WITH STRESS AND FRUSTRATION

When you're caring for others, it's easy to forget to care for yourself. While it may be difficult to find time to focus on yourself and your needs, it is very important that you do so to prevent frustration and burnout.

Caregiving can be rewarding, but also tiring and stressful. Caring for an individual with Alzheimer's disease, dementia, or another health condition is challenging and, at times, overwhelming. Frustration is a normal and valid emotional response to many of the difficulties of being a caregiver. While some irritation may be part of everyday life as a caregiver, feeling extreme frustration can have serious consequences for you or the person you care for. Frustration and stress may negatively impact your physical health or cause you to be physically or verbally aggressive towards your loved one. If your caregiving situation is causing you extreme frustration or anger, you may want to explore some new techniques for coping.

When you are frustrated, it is important to distinguish between *what is and what is not within your power to change*. Frustration often arises out of trying to change an uncontrollable circumstance. If you care for someone with dementia, you face many uncontrollable situations. Normal daily activities—dressing, bathing and eating—may become sources of stress for you. Behaviors often associated with dementia, like wandering or asking questions repeatedly, can be deeply frustrating for caregivers but are uncontrollable behaviors for people with dementia. Unfortunately, you cannot simply change the behavior of a person suffering from dementia.

When dealing with an uncontrollable circumstance, you do control one thing: *how you respond to that circumstance.*

In order to respond without extreme frustration, you will need to

- learn to recognize the warnings signs of stress and frustration;
- intervene to calm yourself down physically;
- modify your thoughts in a way that reduces your stress;
- learn to communicate assertively;
- learn to ask for help.

If you can recognize the warning signs of frustration, you can intervene and adjust your mood before you lose control. Some of the common warning signs of frustration include

- shortness of breath
- knot in the throat
- stomach cramps
- chest pains
- headache
- compulsive eating
- excessive alcohol consumption
- increased smoking
- lack of patience
- desire to strike out

Calming Down Physically

When you become aware of the warning signs of frustration, you can intervene with an immediate activity to help you calm down.

This gives you time to look at the situation more objectively and to choose how to respond in a more controlled way.

When you feel yourself becoming stressed and frustrated, try counting from one to ten slowly and taking a few deep breaths. If you are able, take a brief walk or go to another room and collect your thoughts. It is better to leave the situation, even for a moment, than to lose control or react in a way you will regret. If you think someone may be offended when you leave the room, you can tell that person you need to go to the restroom. You can also try calling a friend, praying, meditating, singing, listening to music or taking a bath. Try experimenting with different responses to find out what works best for you and the person you care for.

The regular practice of relaxation techniques can also help prepare you for frustrating circumstances. If possible, try the following relaxation exercise for at least ten minutes each day:

> Sit in a comfortable position in a quiet place. Take slow, deep breaths and relax the tension in your body. While you continue to take slow, deep breaths, you may want to imagine a safe and restful place and repeat a calming word or phrase.

Modifying Your Thoughts

As you take time out to collect your thoughts, try rethinking your situation in ways that reduce frustration. How you think often affects how you feel. Of course, feelings of stress and frustration arise from difficult circumstances. If, however, you analyze your response to a frustrating situation, you will usually find some form of *maladaptive*—or negative—thinking that has the effect of increasing your frustration, preventing you from looking at your situation objectively, or finding a better way to deal with it.

Below are six major types of unhelpful thought patterns common among caregivers. Following each unhelpful thought pattern is an example of an *adaptive*—or more helpful—thought that can be used as self-defense against frustration. Familiarizing yourself with the unhelpful thought patterns and the adaptive responses can help you control your frustration.

- *Over-generalization:* You take one negative situation or characteristic and multiply it. For example, you're getting ready to take the person in your care to a doctor's appointment when you discover the car battery has died. You then conclude, "This always happens; something always goes wrong."

  Adaptive response: "This does not happen all the time. Usually my car is working just fine. At times things don't happen the way I would like, but sometimes they do."

- *Discounting the positive:* You overlook the good things about your circumstances and yourself. For example, you might not allow yourself to feel good about caregiving by thinking, "I could do more" or "anyone could do what I do."

  Adaptive response: "Caregiving is not easy. It takes courage, strength, and compassion to do what I do. I am not always perfect, but I do a lot and I am trying to be helpful."

- *Jumping to conclusions:* You reach a conclusion without having all the facts. You might do this in two ways:

  - *Mindreading:* We assume that others are thinking negative thoughts about us. For example, a friend doesn't return a phone call, and we assume that he or she is ignoring us or doesn't want to talk to us.

    Adaptive response: "I don't know what my friend is thinking. For all I know, she didn't get the message. Maybe she is busy or just forgot. If I want to know what she is thinking, I will have to ask her."

  - *Fortune-telling:* You predict a negative outcome in the future. For example, you will not try adult day care because you assume the person in your care will not enjoy it. You think, "He will never do that. Not a chance!"

Adaptive response: "I cannot predict the future. I don't think he is going to like it, but I won't know for sure unless I try."

- *"Should" statements:* You try to motivate yourself using statements such as "I should call mother more often" or "I shouldn't go to a movie because Mom might need me." What you think you "should" do is in conflict with what you want to do. You end up feeling guilty, depressed or frustrated.

  Adaptive response: "I would like to go to a movie. It's okay for me to take a break from caregiving and enjoy myself. I will ask a friend or neighbor to check in on Mom."

- *Labeling:* You identify yourself or other people with one characteristic or action. For example, you put off doing the laundry and think, "I am lazy."

  Adaptive response: "I am not lazy. Sometimes I don't do as much as I could, but that doesn't mean I am lazy. I often work hard and do the best that I can. Even I need a break sometimes."

- *Personalizing:* You take responsibility for a negative occurrence that is beyond your control. For example, you might blame yourself when the person in your care requires hospitalization or placement in a facility.

  Adaptive response: "Mom's condition has gotten to the point where I can no longer take care of her myself. It is her condition and not my shortcomings that require her to be in a nursing home."

Using the "Triple-Column" Technique

Unhelpful thought patterns are usually ingrained reactions or habits. To modify your negative thoughts, you will have to learn to recognize them, know why they are false, and talk back to them.

One helpful way to practice using more adaptive thinking processes is to use the "triple-column" technique. Draw two lines down the center of a piece of paper to divide the paper into thirds. When you feel frustrated, take a personal "time out" and write your negative thoughts in the first column.

In the second column, try to identify the type of unhelpful pattern from the six examples above. In the third column, talk back to your negative thoughts with a more positive point of view. See below for examples.

Negative Thoughts	Thought Patterns	Adaptive Thoughts
(Caregiver burns dinner.) "I can't do anything right!"	Over-generalization	I'm not perfect, but nobody is perfect. Sometimes I make mistakes, and sometimes I do things well.
(Caregiver has coffee with a friend and spouse has accident at home.) "I'm selfish and rotten! If I had been home, he wouldn't have fallen."	Labeling; personalizing	I'm not selfish or rotten. I do a lot to take care of my husband, but I need to take care of myself as well. He might have fallen even if I had been home.
(Brother does not show up to take your dad to the doctor.) "I knew I couldn't trust him. I should just do it myself next time."	Jumping to conclusions; "should" statements	I don't know why he didn't come, but I need his help, so we'll have to find ways for him to share the burden of my dad's care.

Communicating Assertively

Good communication can reduce frustration by allowing you to express yourself while helping others to understand your limits and needs. *Assertive* communication is different from passive or aggressive communication. When you communicate passively, you may be keeping your own needs and desires inside to avoid conflict with others. While this may seem easier on the surface, the long-term result may be that others feel they can push you around to get their way.

When you communicate aggressively, you may be forcing your needs and desires onto others. While this allows you to express your feelings, aggressive communication generally makes others more defensive and less cooperative.

When you communicate assertively, you express your own needs and desires while respecting the needs and desires of others. Assertive communication allows both parties to engage in a dignified discussion about the issue at hand.

Keys to assertive communication are:

- Respecting your own feelings, needs, and desires.
- Standing up for your feelings without shaming, degrading or humiliating the other person.
- Using "I" statements rather than "You" statements. For example, say, "I need a break" or "I would like to talk to you and work this out" instead of "You are irresponsible" or "You never help out!"
- Not using "should" statements. For example, say, "It's important to me that promises be kept," instead of "You should keep your promise."

The Critical Step: Asking for Help

You cannot take on all the responsibilities of caregiving by yourself. It is essential that you ask for and accept help. Discuss your needs with family members and friends who might be willing to share caregiving responsibilities. People will not realize you need help if you do not explain your situation and ask for assistance. Remember, you have the right to ask for help and express your needs.

When to Say "Yes"

Don't be afraid to say "Yes" if someone offers to help. Say "Yes" at the moment a person offers to help rather than saying "Maybe" and waiting until you are in a fix. Have a list handy of errands or tasks you need help with. Keep in mind that people feel useful and gratified when they are able to help others.

When to Say "No"

Often caregivers are pulled in multiple directions. In addition to the demands of caregiving, you may feel compelled to meet the demands of your immediate and extended family, your friends, and your employer. Learn how to say "No" to the demands of others when you are overwhelmed or need a break. It is your right to say "No" to extra demands on your time without feeling guilty.

Learning Effective Communication Techniques

Many families find it especially frustrating to communicate with a loved one who has dementia. The person with dementia may repeat questions over and over or mistake you for someone else. It is important to remember that persons with dementia cannot control behavior caused by their disease. They do not need to be corrected or grounded in "reality." You can distract them or just agree with them as a way to reduce your frustration.

It can be helpful, however, to learn more about dementia and effective communication techniques, which will ease your frustration. For example, use simple, direct statements and place yourself close when speaking to a person with a cognitive disorder. Try not to argue about unimportant things such as what the date is. Allow extra time to accomplish tasks such as dressing. Remember, people with dementia often react more to our feelings than our words. Finding ways to be calm can help you to gain cooperation. See the Family Caregiver Alliance Fact Sheet:

Caregiver's Guide to Understanding Dementia Behaviors at <http:// caregiver.org/caregiver/jsp/content_node.jsp?nodeid=391> for more helpful strategies.

Taking Care of *You*

Although caregiving may make it difficult to find time for yourself, it is important to eat well, exercise, get a good night's sleep and attend to your own medical needs.

When you do not take care of yourself, you are prone to increased anxiety, depression, frustration and physical distress that will make it more difficult to continue providing care.

Make Time for Yourself

You may feel guilty about needing or wanting time out for rest, socialization, and fun. However, everyone deserves regular and ongoing breaks from work, including caregivers. "Respite" providers can give you the opportunity to take the breaks you need. Respite breaks may be provided by in-home help, adult day care, "friendly visitor" programs, relatives, friends, and neighbors, or other means. The important point is to allow yourself to take a break from caregiving. See "Resources" at the end of this section for organizations that might help you give yourself time off from caregiving.

Seek Outside Support

Sharing your feelings with a counselor, a pastor, a support group, or another caregiver in a similar situation can be a great way to release stress and get helpful advice. You may want to contact the organizations under "Resources" at the end of this chapter or look in the community services section at the front of the *Yellow Pages,* under "Counseling" or "Senior Services" to find services to help you get some caregiver support. The Family Caregiver Alliance Fact Sheet on Community Care Options at <http://caregiver.org/caregiver/jsp/content_node.jsp?nodeid =394> also offers information.

Credits

Burns, David. (1980, 1999). *Feeling Good: The New Mood Therapy.* Revised and updated edition. New York: Avon Books.

Gallagher-Thompson, D., et al. (1992). *Controlling Your Frustration: A Class for Caregivers.* Palo Alto, CA: Department of Veterans Affairs Medical Center.

Parrish, Monique. (2000). *"Stress: What Is It? What Can Be Done About It?" Stress Reduction Instruction Manual,* written for John Muir Mount Diablo Medical Center, Concord, CA.

Resources

Family Caregiver Alliance National Center on Caregiving
180 Montgomery Street, Suite 1100
San Francisco, CA 94104
(415) 434-3388
(800) 445-8106 (toll free)
Website: www.caregiver.org
Email: info@caregiver.org

Family Caregiver Alliance (FCA) seeks to improve the quality of life for caregivers through education, services, research, and advocacy.

Through its National Center on Caregiving, FCA offers information on current social, public policy, and caregiving issues and provides assistance in the development of public and private programs and in locating support services for family caregivers.

For residents of the greater San Francisco Bay Area, FCA provides information, education, and direct support services for caregivers of those with Alzheimer's disease, stroke, traumatic brain injury, Parkinson's and other debilitating disorders that strike adults.

Helpful Family Caregiver Alliance Fact Sheets:

Caregiver's Guide to Understanding Dementia Behaviors

http://caregiver.org/caregiver/jsp/content_node.jsp?nodeid
=391

Hiring In-Home Help
http://caregiver.org/caregiver/jsp/content_node.
jsp?nodeid=407

Taking Care of YOU: Self-Care for Family Caregivers
http://caregiver.org/caregiver/jsp/content_node.
jsp?nodeid=847

Alzheimer's Association
225 N. Michigan Ave., Ste. 1700
Chicago, IL 60601-7633
(800) 272-3900
www.alz.org

Eldercare Locator
Call to find your local Area Agency on Aging and services for
the elderly and caregivers, including respite care providers.
(800) 677-1116
www.eldercare.gov

Faith in Action
Call to find volunteer caregiving assistance.
(877) 324-8411 (toll-free)
www.fiavolunteers.org

ARCH National Respite Network and Resource Center
Call to find local respite providers.
(919) 490-5577
www.archrespite.org/index.htm

Prepared by Family Caregiver Alliance. Funded by the California Department of Mental Health. ©2003 Family Caregiver Alliance. Used with permission.